Fibroids

Edited by Hassan Abduljabbar

Published in London, United Kingdom

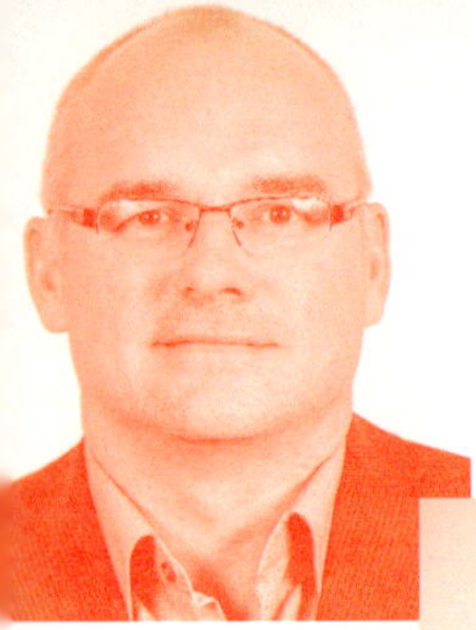
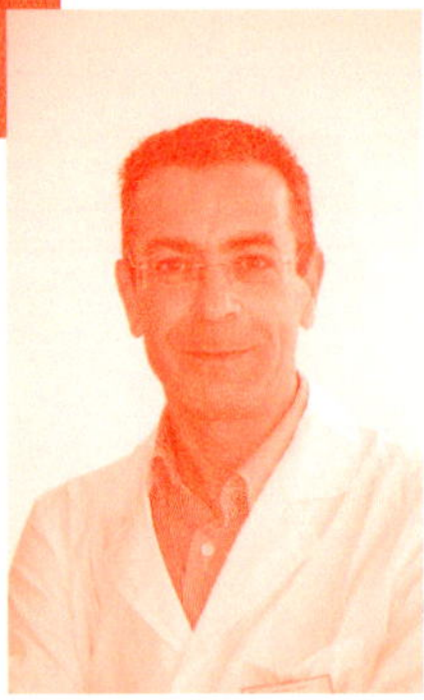
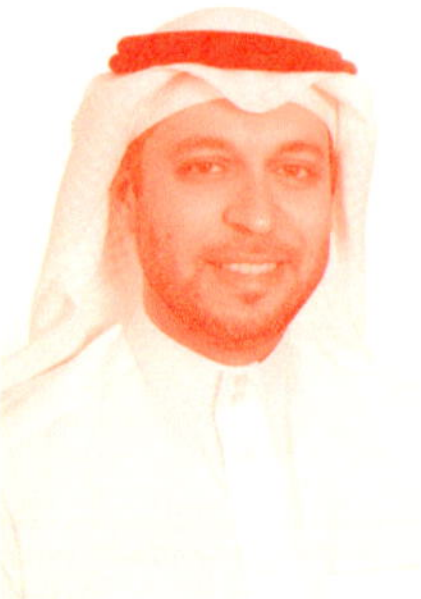
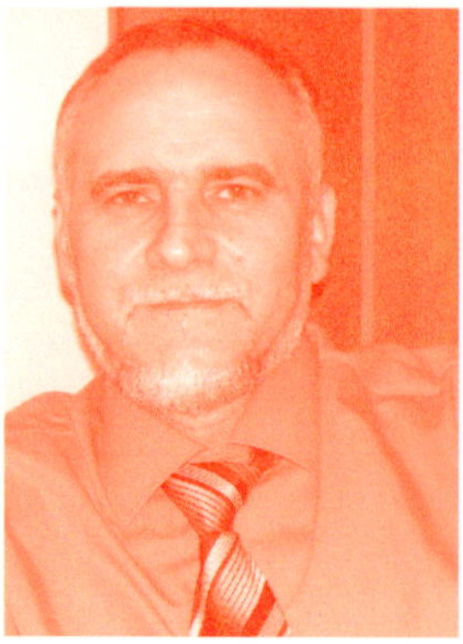
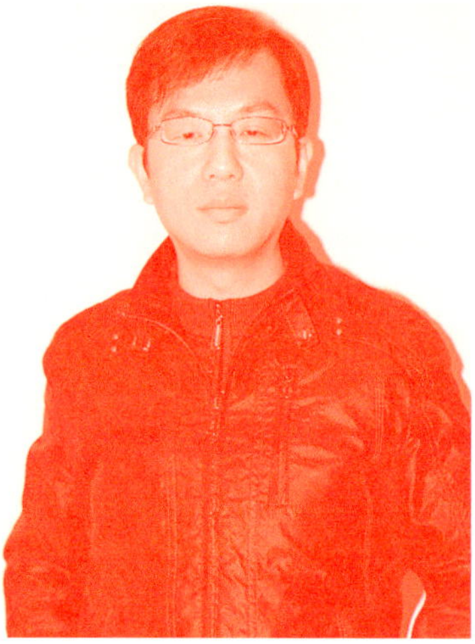
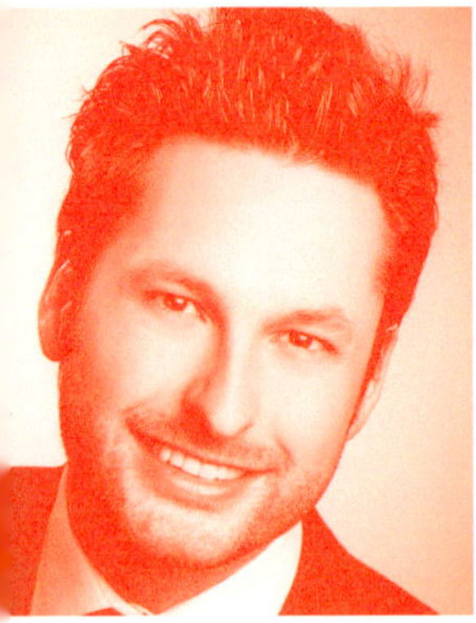
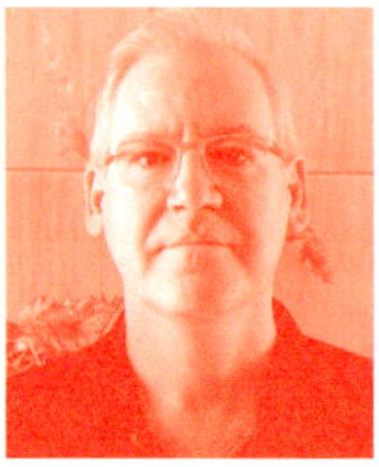

IntechOpen

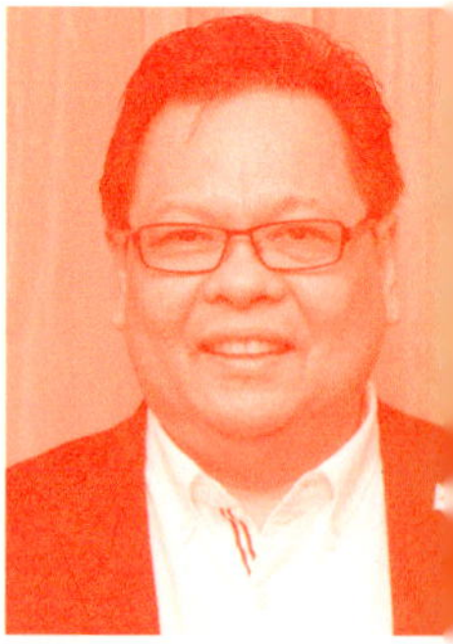
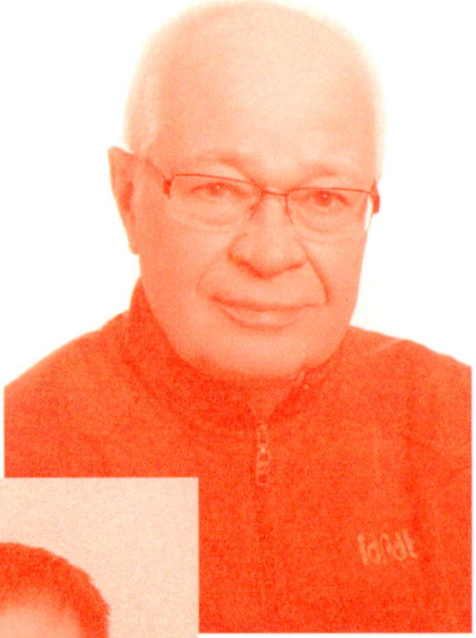
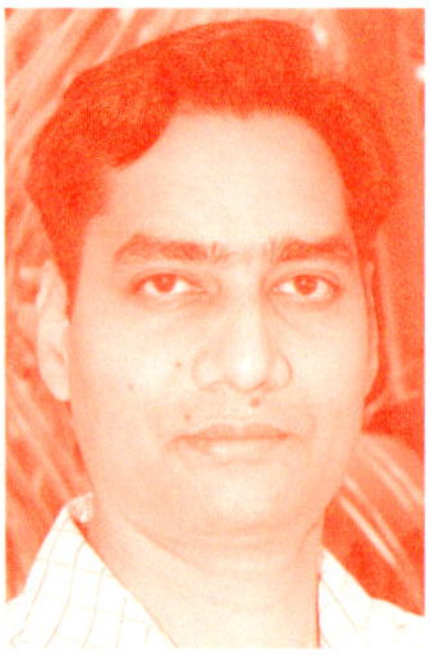
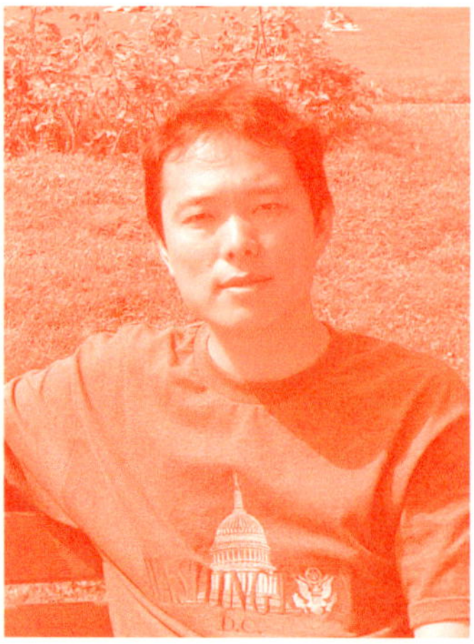
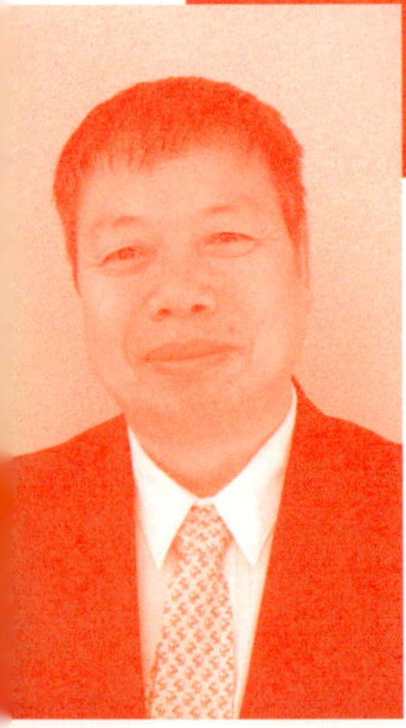
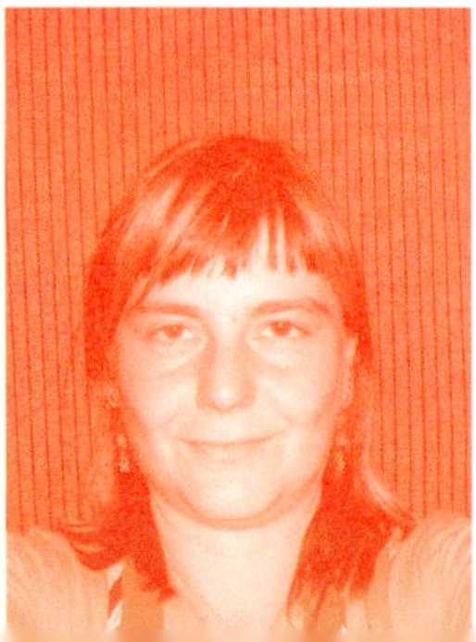

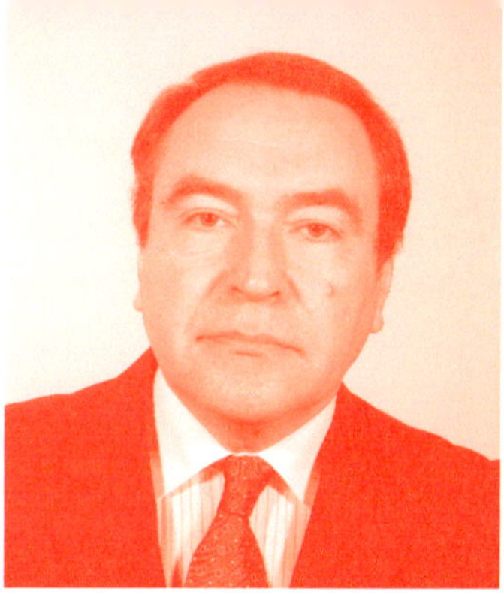

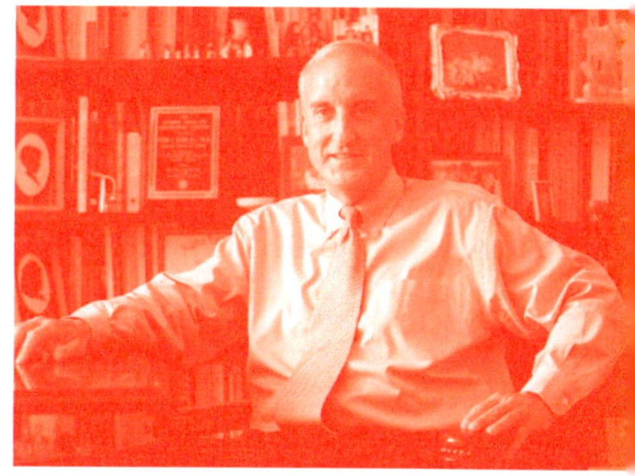

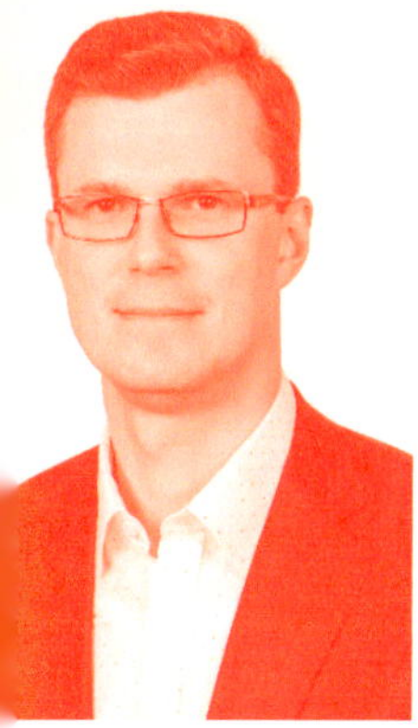

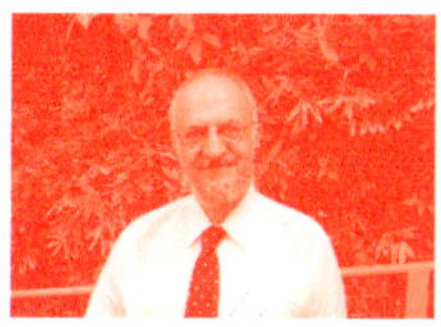

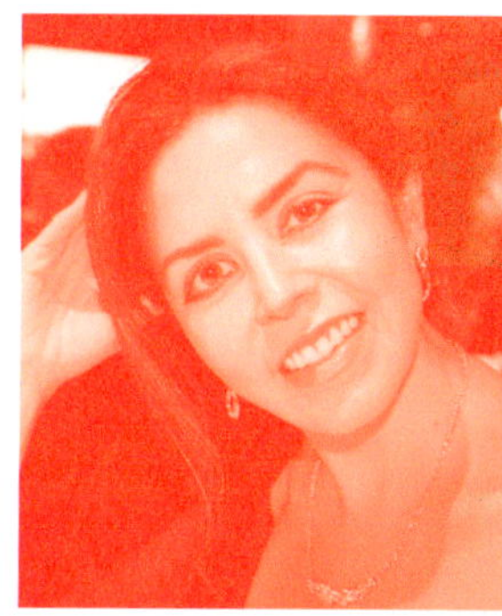

Supporting open minds since 2005

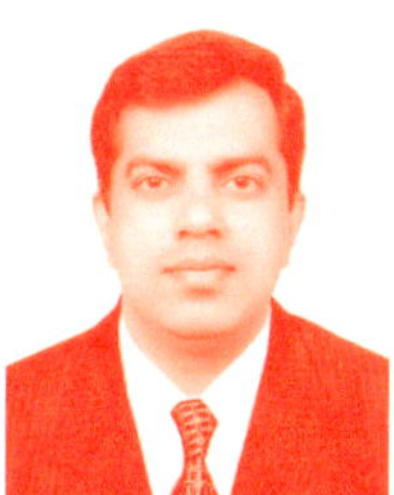

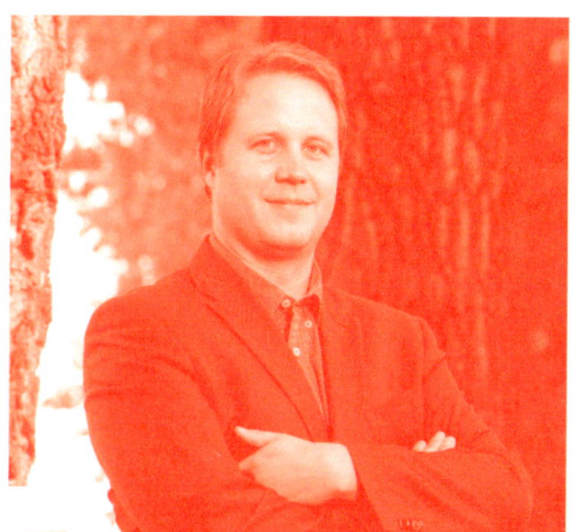

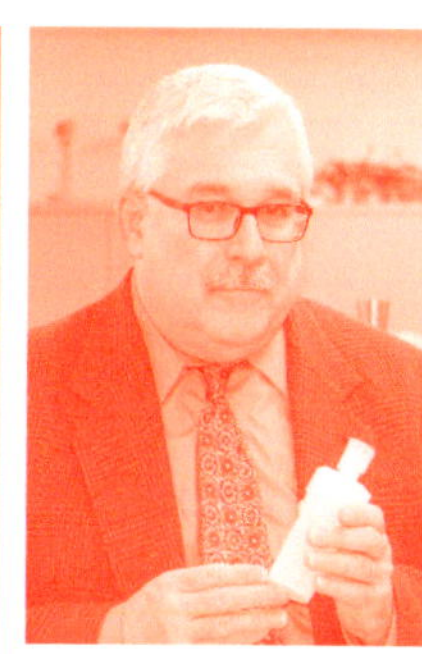

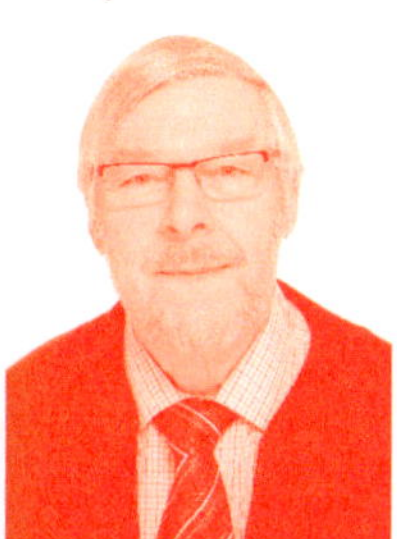

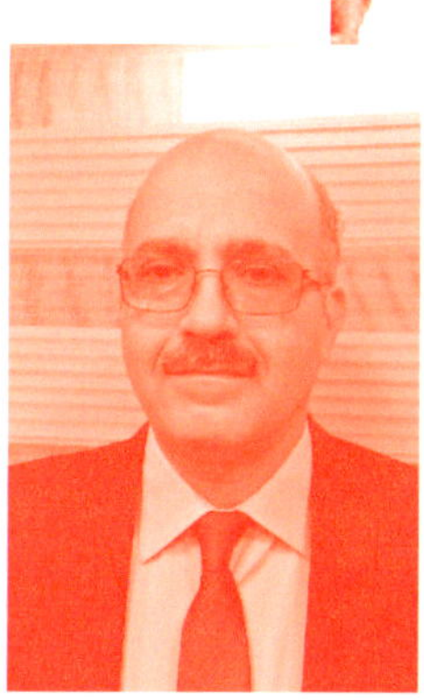

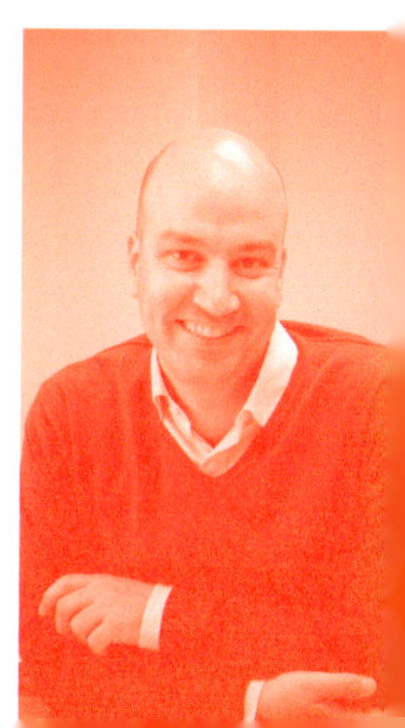

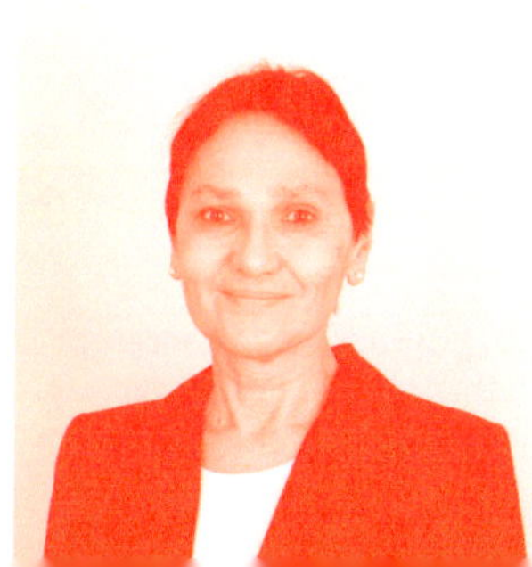

Fibroids
http://dx.doi.org/10.5772/intechopen.92500
Edited by Hassan Abduljabbar

Contributors
Havagiray R. Chitme, Joel Noutakdie Tochie, Gregory Ayissi, Julius Dohbit Sama, Sergio Rosales-Ortiz, Jose Fugarolas Marin, Tammy Barrón Martinez, Diana Sulvaran Victoria, Jocelyn Arias Alarcon, Janeth Marquez-Acosta, Panagiotis Tsikouras, Anastasia Bothou, Xanthoula Anthoulaki, Rakesh Gupta, Poonam Wasnik, eman alshawish, Hung-Yun Lin, Zi-Lin Li, Tung-Yung Huang, Yih Ho, Ya-Jung Shih, Yi-Ru Chen, Heng-Yuan Tang, Jaqueline Whang-Peng, Kuan Wang, Cinta Vidal Mazo, Kizito Omona, Pankaj Pant, Anna Chalkidou, Spyridon Michalopoulos, Nistikoulis George, Ioannis Tsirkas, Fotini Gaitatzi, Selma Gyroglou, Irene Babageorgaka, Natalia Sachnova, Michael Koutsogiannis, Apostolos Lazarou, Arsou Chalil Bouratzan, Theopi Nalbanti, Panagiotis Peitsidis, Konstantinos Nikolettos, George Dragoutsos, Thedosia Vogaitzaki, Stefanos Zervoudis, George Iatrakis, Werner Rath, Nikolaos Nikolettos, Vasileios Souftas, Gaelle Therese Badjang

First published in London, United Kingdom, 2021 by IntechOpen
IntechOpen is the global imprint of INTECHOPEN LIMITED, registered in England and Wales, registration number: 11086078, 5 Princes Gate Court, London, SW7 2QJ, United Kingdom
Printed in Croatia

British Library Cataloguing-in-Publication Data
A catalogue record for this book is available from the British Library

Additional hard and PDF copies can be obtained from orders@intechopen.com

Fibroids
Edited by Hassan Abduljabbar
p. cm.
Print ISBN 978-1-83962-995-2
Online ISBN 978-1-83962-996-9
eBook (PDF) ISBN 978-1-83968-011-3

Meet the editor

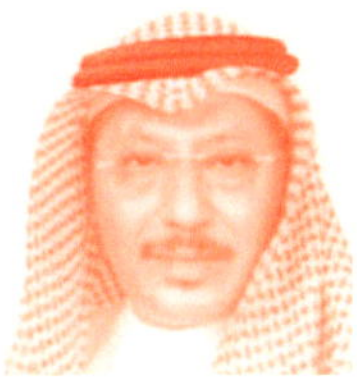

Hassan S. Abduljabbar, MD, FRCSC, is Professor of Obstetrics and Gynecology, King Abdulaziz University, Jeddah, Saudi Arabia. He is president of the Saudi Society of Obstetrics and Gynecology and the Federation of Arab Gynecology Obstetrics Societies. Dr. Abduljabbar graduated from King Abdulaziz University in 1980 and the University of Western Ontario in 1986. He was board certified by the American Board of Obstetrics and Gynecology (ABOG) in 1988. He is a reviewer for many international scientific journals and an examiner of master's degrees and Ph.D.'s as well as for the Saudi and Arab board exams. He has published seventy-five articles and edited several books. He also writes on scientific subjects for local newspapers like Al-Bilad.

Contents

Preface

This important book explores one of the most common pathologic abnormalities of the female genital tract: fibroids. A fibroid is a benign tumor originating from the smooth muscle of the uterus.

Written by authors and researchers in the field, this book examines uterine fibroids over four sections. The first section covers the clinical presentation of myoma. Some tumors are asymptomatic, whereas others may cause pelvic masses, abnormal vaginal bleeding, or pelvic pain. It also discusses sexual dysfunction as well as reproductive symptoms like infertility and recurrent pregnancy loss.

The second section deals with the diagnosis, which can be accomplished by conducting a clinical history and physical examination, including pelvic examination. Diagnosis can be confirmed via pelvic ultrasound, computed tomography (CT) scan, or magnetic resonance imaging (MRI), all of which can also be used to diagnose extra-uterine fibroids as well. This section includes a chapter about submucous myoma and hysteroscopy and how the latter can treat bleeding in uterine myxomatosis.

The third section deals with the management of uterine fibroids, including medical hormonal or non-hormonal treatment, herbal medicine, surgery (either open or endoscopic), and uterine artery embolization. It also discusses women's perspectives about their bodies after hysterectomy.

Hassan Abduljabbar
Department of Obstetrics and Gynecology,
King Abdulaziz University,
Jeddah, Saudi Arabia

Section 1

Clinical Presentation

Chapter 1

Bleeding

Kizito Omona

Abstract

Fibroid, also called leiomyomas, is common tumor of the uterus. Usually, women of reproductive age are at risk of getting it. However, majority of these women develop fibroid (s) by the age of 50 years. This condition usually causes painful and unpleasant symptoms such as; heavy bleeding, prolonged periods, inter-menstrual bleeding, abdominal pain and cramps, anemia, pelvic pain and pain during sexual intercourse, among others. Abnormal bleeding, such as bleeding that occurs with fibroids and heavy periods, often lasts more than 10 days per month. This fibroid symptom involves persistent bleeding between cycles, which can severely impact one's quality of life. Abnormal bleeding, especially in fibroids, can be taken as missing three or more periods in a woman who had been having regular monthly period, or periods that last less than 21 days or more than 35 days apart from each other. Another indication of an abnormal period is bleeding through multiple pads and tampons in a short amount of time.

Keywords: per vaginal bleeding, abnormal bleeding, normal bleeding, menstrual bleeding, menstrual cycle

1. Introduction

In a normal adult human – female, menstrual cycle occurs to provide for release of oocyte, thus preparing the uterus for any possible pregnancy [1].

Thus, menstruation is a woman's normal monthly per vaginal bleeding, usually called "monthly period." When a woman menstruates, her body discards the monthly build-up of the lining of the uterus. The resultant blood, also called menstrual blood, and uterine tissues flow from the uterus through the cervix and then into the vagina and eventually out of the body [2]. In other words, menstruation is the cyclic and orderly sloughing off of the uterine lining which occurs in response to the interactions of hormones produced by the hypothalamus, pituitary and ovaries [3].

Menstrual cycle is, thus, divided into three phases. These are follicular or proliferative phase, ovulation and luteal or secretory phase. The number of days between the first day of menstrual bleeding of a woman's cycle to the onset of menses of the next cycle is referred to as 'the length of a menstrual cycle'. The average duration of a menstrual cycle is usually 28 days. However, some women may have shorter cycle of 21 days. Such women are referred to as 'polymenorrheic women'. Some women also have longer cycle of 35 days or more. These are called oligomenorrheic women [3]. Thus, the complete cycle may last anywhere from 21 days to 35 days with an average duration of 28 days for most women.

Menstruation begins at puberty, usually between ranging 10 to 16 years of age of a normal girl child. It ends at menopause, corresponding to average age of 45 to 55 years of a normal adult female [1].

Ordinarily, the typical volume of blood lost during menstruation is approximately 30 milliliters (mL). Any amount of blood lost during menstruation which is greater than 80 mL is considered abnormal [4].

2. Physiology of normal uterine bleeding

There are four major circulating hormones involved in the menstrual cycle. These hormones are; follicle stimulating hormones (FSH), luteinizing hormones (LH), estradiol (estrogen) and progesterone. The concentrations of these hormones in blood vary and their levels provide characteristic changes during the menstrual cycle [5]. In particular, the body makes three main types of estrogen; estrone (E1), estradiol (E2) and estriol (E3). E1 is the only estrogen the body makes after menopause. E2 is the most common type in women of childbearing age whereas E3 is the main estrogen during pregnancy [6].

The menstrual cycle is triggered by the gonadotropin-releasing hormone (GnRH) pulse generator in the hypothalamus. The GnRH pulse generator then releases gonadotropin-releasing hormone (GnRH) [7]. This GnRH in turn stimulates the synthesis and release of the gonadotropins, luteinizing hormones (LH) and follicle stimulating hormones (FSH), from the anterior pituitary gland [5]. LH and FSH exert their effects in the ovaries. There are two types of cells responsible for hormone production within the ovarian follicle; theca cells and granulosa cells. LH acts on theca cells to produce progesterone and androstenedione. The enzyme involved is cholesterol desmolase. Upon secretion of androstenedione, the hormone diffuses to granulosa cells. FSH then stimulates the granulosa cells to convert androstenedione to testosterone and eventually 17-beta-estradiol. The enzyme involved is aromatase. The levels of 17-beta-estradiol or progesterone increases accordingly, depending on the phase of the menstrual cycle. This increase triggers a negative feedback back to the anterior pituitary to lower the levels of FSH and LH which are being produced and subsequently, the levels of 17-beta-estradiol and progesterone produced. The only exception occurs during ovulation, in which case, once a critical amount of 17-beta-estradiol is produced it provides positive feedback to the anterior pituitary instead of a negative feedback [5, 6]. This positive feedback results in increased amounts of FSH and LH, hence the LH surge bringing about ovulation [1].

The onset of the menstrual cycle, or menarche, usually at 10–16 years, begins at puberty and ceases at menopause, usually 45–55 years. The cycle has 3 phases: follicular or proliferative phase, ovulation and luteal or secretory phase [1, 5].

Follicular Phase: Usually, the first phase of the menstrual cycle is the follicular or proliferative phase. The phase is characterized by menstruation, resulting from shedding off of the initially thickened endometrial lining following failed fertilization or implantation. It occurs from day zero to day 14 of the menstrual cycle (see **Figures 1** and **2**), based on the average duration of 28 days cycle. There is usually variability in the length of menstrual cycle and this is due to variations in the length of the follicular phase. The main hormone during this phase is estrogen, in particular 17-beta-estradiol [1, 5] from the ovary coupled with follicle stimulating hormone (FSH), released from anterior pituitary gland. Upon release from anterior pituitary, FSH and LH slowly rise in levels and cause the growth of follicles on the surface of the ovary. This process prepares the egg for ovulation. As the follicles grow, they begin releasing estrogens and a low level of progesterone. These ovarian hormones then inhibit further release of GnRH from the hypothalamus, in a

DOI: http://dx.doi.org/10.5772/intechopen.94079

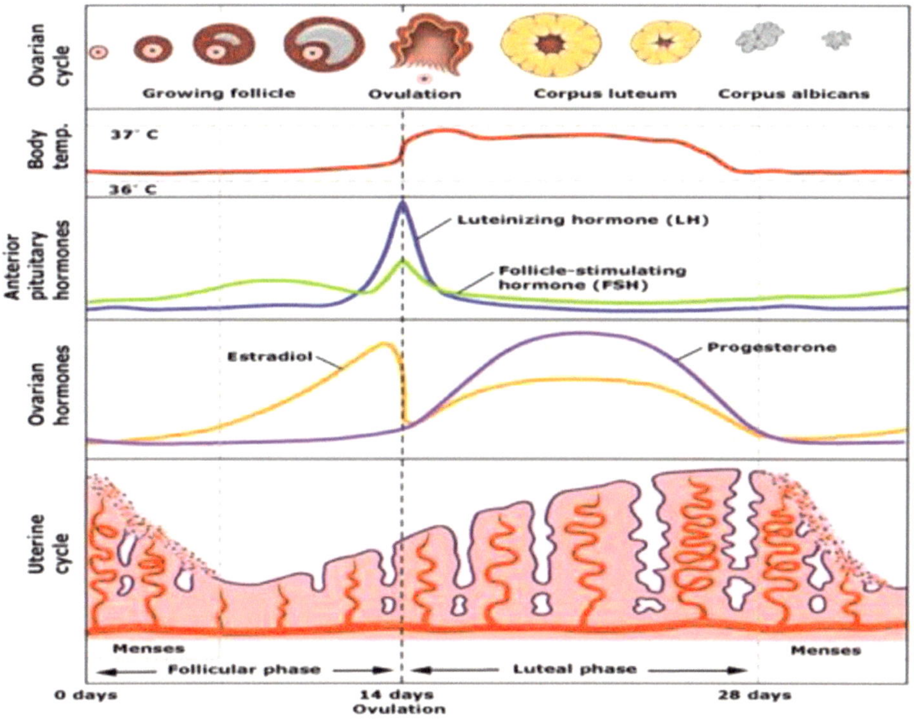

Figure 1.
Hormonal changes in the menstrual cycle.

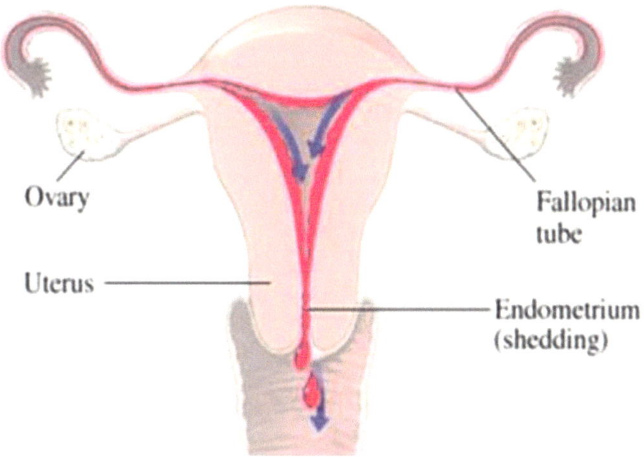

Figure 2.
Menstrual flow.

negative feedback process (See **Figure 3**). Thus, as the follicular phase progresses to the end, the increased amounts of 17-beta-estradiol will provide negative feedback to the anterior pituitary.

Due to the rise of FSH during the first days of the menstrual cycle or follicular phase, several ovarian follicles are stimulated. These ovarian follicles compete with each other for dominance. The follicle that reaches maturity is called a Graafian follicle. During follicular phase, estrogen suppresses production of luteinizing hormone (LH) from the pituitary gland (**Figures 4** and **5**) [5].

Ovulation phase: Ovulation phase comes next. Ovulation occurs 14 days later after the first day of menstruation [1]. This means that with an average 28-day cycle, ovulation occurs on day 14 (see **Figure 1**).

At the end of the proliferative phase, 17-beta-estradiol (E2) levels are high due to the follicle maturation. During the follicular phase, estrogen suppresses production of luteinizing hormone (LH) from the pituitary gland but in this phase it stimulates

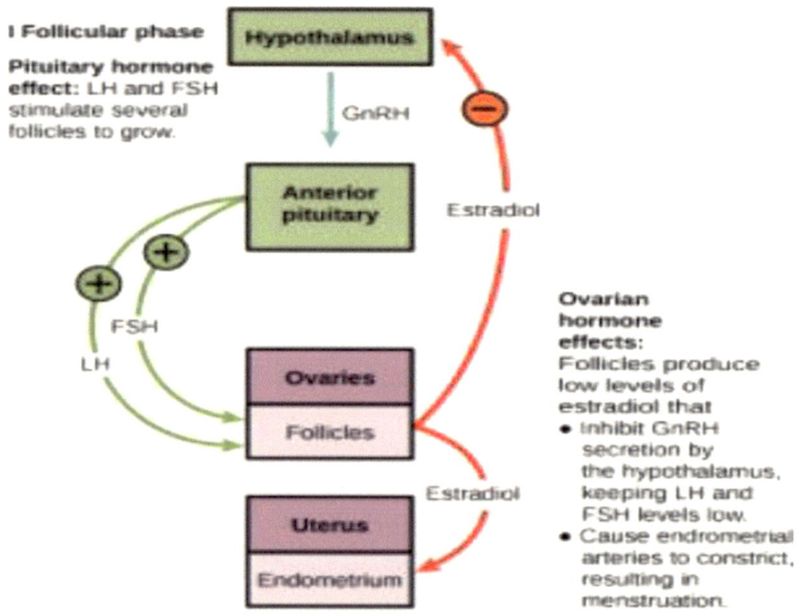

Figure 3.
The follicular phase [5].

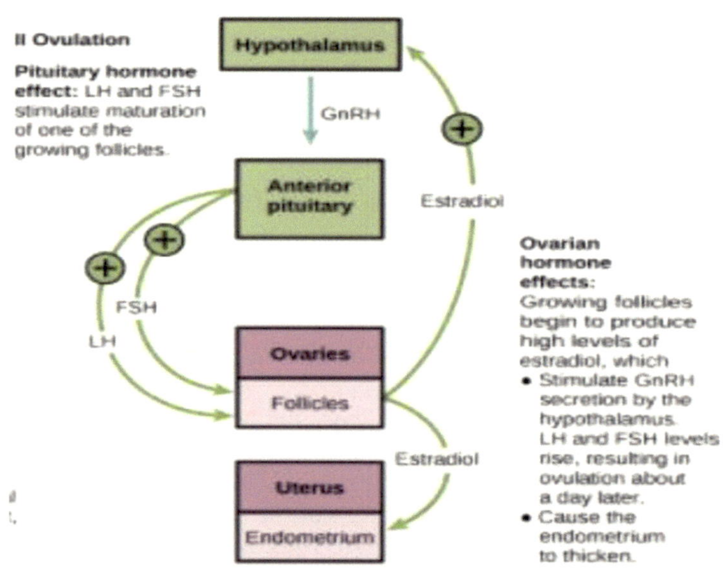

Figure 4.
The ovulation phase [5].

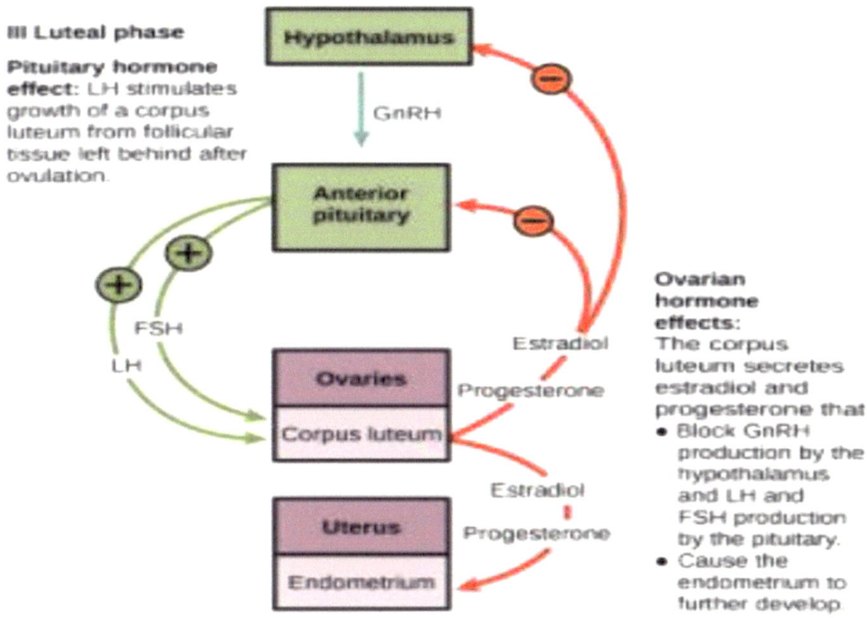

Figure 5.
The luteal phase [5].

maturation a follicle and thickens the endometrial lining. At this time, only 17-beta-estradiol (E2) provides positive feedback for FSH and LH production. A critical level of 17-beta-estradiol must be reached, at least 200 picograms per milliliter of plasma, to cause this positive feedback. The high levels of FSH and LH present during this time is called the LH surge [5]. The release of LH matures the ovum much further and weakens the wall of the follicle in the ovary, thus causing the fully developed follicle to release its secondary oocyte, in a process known as ovulation. After being released from the ovary, the ovum, also called egg, is swept into the fallopian tube.

The changes to the cervix which was initiated during the follicular phase is even further increased in ovulation phase allowing for increased, waterier cervical mucus in order to better accommodate the possible sperm. The levels of 17-beta-estradiol fall at the end of ovulation [1, 5, 6].

Luteal or Secretory phase: The luteal phase follows ovulation. It is characterized by the development of corpus luteum, secretion of progesterone and the formation of thick mucus which blocks the cervix. Blocking of the cervix is in anticipation that implantation has occurred [5]. Luteal phase always occurs from day 14 to day 28 of the cycle (See **Figure 1**). Progesterone stimulated by LH is the dominant hormone during this phase to prepare the corpus luteum and the endometrium for possible implantation of the fertilized ovum. As the luteal phase comes to an end, progesterone will provide negative feedback to the anterior pituitary to decrease FSH and LH levels and subsequently, the 17-beta-estradiol (E2) and progesterone levels [1, 5, 6].

Therefore, at the end of luteal phase, in the absence of implantation (pregnancy), when the level of progesterone drops, menses or menstruation occurs [1]. See **Figure 2**.

3. Clinical significance of physiology of normal uterine bleeding

A normal woman has an average of 450 menses throughout her lifetime. It is therefore, very important to fully understand the menstrual cycle and its physiology as various complications may occur later in life for a woman [8]. The knowledge of this forms the cornerstone of making appropriate diagnosis and investigation [9].

Menstruation begins at puberty, usually between 10 to 16 years of age of a normal girl child. It ends at menopause, corresponding to average age of 45 to 55 years of a normal adult female [1].

Ordinarily, the typical volume of blood lost during menstruation is approximately 30 milliliters (mL). Any amount of blood lost during menstruation which is greater than 80 mL is considered abnormal [4].

The clinician needs to know all these in order to make appropriate diagnosis and investigation. Anything sort of this could result in gross errors.

4. Bleeding in fibroids

Fibroids are growths of muscle and fibrous tissue in or on the wall of the uterus.

They range in size from seedlings which are undetectable by human eye, to bulky masses that can disfigure or enlarge the uterus. One can have a single fibroid or multiple fibroids (See **Figure 6**) [10].

4.1 Normal versus abnormal bleeding

It is usually very difficult to tell between what is normal and what is abnormal when it comes to menstruation. This is because of the huge variation in women to the point that what is normal for one might be abnormal for another. Heavy menstrual flow is highly subjective.

In addition to the above, there are many factors that influence length, heaviness, and frequency of a woman's menstrual flow. Thus, paying close attention to one's monthly period and observing the trend becomes paramount to detecting whether or not one has abnormal or normal menstrual flow. This observance might need to have been done over a significant period of time [11].

Vaginal bleeding is considered to be abnormal if it occurs between a woman's menstrual cycles, in situations where flow is significantly heavier than normal for a particular individual or when it occurs after menopause.

4.1.1 Normal bleeding

Bleeding in normal period typically lasts between 3 and 8 days, usually with a heavier menstrual flow for the first two days. The flow gets increasingly lighter as

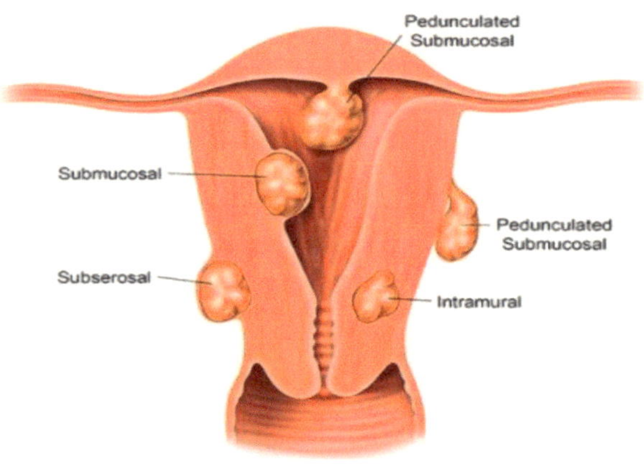

Figure 6.
Different locations of fibroids [10].

the number of days progress. Women with normal periods may have limited spotting, cramps that ache and bloating that goes away once the period is over.

4.1.2 Abnormal periods or fibroids bleeding

On another hand, abnormal bleeding, such as those bleedings occurring in fibroids and in heavy periods, usually lasts more than 10 days per month. Fibroid symptom involves persistent bleeding between menstrual cycles. This is to the point that can severely affect one's quality of life [11].

Abnormal bleeding can be considered missing 3 or more periods in a row, or periods which occur less than 21 days or more than 35 days apart from each other. Another sign of an abnormal period is bleeding through multiple pads and tampons in a short amount of time [10, 11].

4.2 The cause of heavy bleeding in fibroids

The cause of heavy bleeding in fibroid is not well understood. Since fibroids are connected to your uterine lining, the fibroids can exert pressure against the uterine wall and cause the endometrial tissue to bleed more than normal [11]. See **Figure 6.**

During menstrual period, the uterine lining sheds off and the uterus has two basic mechanisms to stop itself from bleeding. The first mechanism is through the normal blood-clotting working throughout the body by forming plugs within the blood vessels. Secondly, since the uterus is a muscle, it also has the ability to contract the bleeding vessels of the uterus, thus stopping the bleeding. The contractions are associated with menstrual cramps.

However, it is believed that fibroids interfere with adequate and proper contraction of the uterus. In this way, it does not stop menstrual bleeding adequately. Additionally, fibroids produce growth factors (proteins) that stimulate relaxation of the uterine blood vessels and thus causing more blood in the uterine cavity, which leads to heavier periods [11].

4.3 Treatment of abnormal bleeding and fibroids bleeding

The treatment of abnormal bleeding depend on; the cause, patient age, severity of bleeding and whether one wants to have children or not [12].

Otherwise, the common medical treatment options are;

1. Use of birth control pills

2. Hormone injections or a hormone-releasing IUD (intra-uterine device)

3. Surgery to control bleeding or to remove growths, such as fibroids, that are causing the bleeding. Surgical options available include endometrial ablation, endometrial polyp removal, myomectomy or even hysterectomy

The two medical treatments for heavy menstrual bleeding have been effective enough. First, levonorgestrel intra-uterine system was FDA approved for the treatment of heavy menstrual bleeding in 2009. It is highly effective for decreasing menstrual bleeding, treating anemia and improving the overall quality of life. Secondly, tranexamic acid, also FDA approved for heavy menstrual bleeding in 2009, reduces menstrual blood loss in 40% of women and improves quality of life. Moreover, in women with fibroids, tranexamic acid has been shown to decrease heavy menstrual bleeding and cause necrosis of the fibroids, especially larger fibroids [13].

5. Conclusion

Research on bleeding in fibroids is still far from over. Much more is still wanting.

Uterine fibroids are common debilitating problems for many women. Almost 60% of women with fibroids report that symptoms affect their quality of life and impede their physical activity. Again, 24% of them report that fibroid symptoms prevent them from reaching their full potential at work. Heavy menstrual bleeding, which is the most common symptom of uterine fibroids, affects approximately 1.4 million women per year.

Acknowledgements

I do acknowledge the technical guidance of my colleagues in the Faculty of Health Sciences of Uganda Martyrs' University. In a special way I appreciate Ms. Scovia Mbabazi, the former Associate Dean and Mr. Mathias Lwenge, the current Associate Dean at the faculty.

Conflict of interest

The author declares no conflict of interest.

Author details

Kizito Omona
Uganda Martyrs University, Faculty of Health Sciences, Kampala, Uganda

*Address all correspondence to: komona@umu.ac.ug

References

[1] Thiyagarajan, D. K., Basit, H. and Jeanmonod, R. Physiology, *Menstrual Cycle.* Treasure Island(FL) : StatPearls Publishing, 2020.

[2] Office on Women's Health [OWH]. What is Menstruation? *Womenshealth. gov.* [Online] 2018. https://www.womenshealth.gov/menstrual-cycle/your-menstrual-cycle.

[3] Reed, B. G. and Carr, B. R. *The Normal Menstrual Cycle and the Control of Ovulation.* Texas : Endotext, 2018. NBK279054.

[4] Hallberg, L., et al. Menstrual blood loss--a population study. Variation at different ages and attempts to define normality. *Acta Obstet Gynecol Scand.* 1966. Vol. 45, 3, pp. 320-351.

[5] Anon. Hormonal Control of Human Reproduction. [book auth.] C. Molnar and J. Gair. *Concept of Biology- 1st Canadian Edition.* Ottawa : BCcampus, 2019.

[6] Hormone Health Network. Hormone Health Network."Estrogen | Hormone Health Network" . *Hormone.org.* [Online] 2020. https://www.hormone.org/your-health-and-hormones/glands-and-hormones-a-to-z/hormones/estrogen.

[7] Ferin, M. *The Hypothalamic-Hypophyseal-Ovarian Axis and the Menstrual Cycle.* New York : Global Library of Women's Medicine, 2008.

[8] Alvergne, A. and Jun, Högqvist, T. V. Is Female Health Cyclical? Evolutionary Perspectives on Menstruation. *Trends Ecol. Evol. (Amst.).* 2018. Vol. 33, 6, pp. 399-414.

[9] Gunn, H. M., et al. Menstrual Patterns in the First Gynecological Year: A Systematic Review. *J Pediatr Adolesc Gynecol.* 2018. Vol. 31, 6, pp. 557-565.

[10] Azura Vascular Care. Could I Be Bleeding Due to Fibroids? *azuravascularcare.com.* [Online] 2018. https://www.azuravascularcare.com/infoufe/bleeding-due-to-fibroids/.

[11] USA Fibroids Centre. DO FIBROIDS CAUSE HEAVY BLEEDING? *usafibroidcentre.com.* [Online] 2020. https://www.usafibroidcenters.com/blog/fibroids-cause-heavy-menstrual-bleeding/.

[12] Anon. Uterine Fibroids & Abnormal Bleeding. *umwomenshealth.org.* [Online] n.d. https://www.umwomenshealth.org/conditions-treatments/uterine-fibroids-abnormal-bleeding.

[13] Laughlin-Tommaso, S. K. and Clinic, Mayo. Treatment of Heavy Menstrual Bleeding in Women With Uterine Fibroids. *ClinicalTrials.gov.* [Online] 2020. https://clinicaltrials.gov/ct2/show/NCT03317795.

Chapter 2

Inflammation and Ovulation

Pankaj Pant and Havagiray R. Chitme

Abstract

The ovulation is a complex physiological process which is very commonly affected in patients with PCOS. Understanding inflammatory process involved in ovulation is important with respect to its onset, diagnosis and treatment. There are multiple inflammatory factors are associated with ovulation however anovulation and contraception have not been therapeutically explored in context with inflammatory process. Therefore, this chapter is written to help readers to understand the basics of inflammation in ovulation and role of inflammatory mediators in ovulation. This chapter also describes genetic and molecular aspects linked to ovulation.

Keywords: inflammation, ovulation, cytokine, prostaglandin, TNF-alpha, PPAR-γ

1. Introduction

Mammalian ovulation is a fundamental physiological process involves the rupturing of follicle and releasing of the dominant follicle from the ovary into the fallopian tube where it has the potential to get fertilized if it exposed to sperm. Oocyte is covered up of four different layers namely the granulosa cells, which form a protected layer within oocyte and the extra follicular microenvironment, then theca layers of theca-interna and theca-externa, tunica albuginea and the outermost one is epithelium [1, 2]. A thin transparent layer between oocyte and follicular membrane is made up of secretions by the oocyte, termed as zona pellucida [2].

The developing oocyte enclosed in a ovarian follicle which is float in a dynamic fluid i.e. Follicular fluid (FF), contain variety of signaling molecules such as polysaccharides, hormones, cytokines, chemokines, growth factors, reactive oxygen species (ROS), metabolites, antioxidant enzymes, etc. The follicular fluid formed in developing antral follicles, primarily to support the development and protection of oocytes. These molecules are also acts as communicators between somatic and germ cells [3].

The duration of ovulatory process in humans, pigs, rats and rabbits takes approximately 40, 22, 12 and 10 hours respectively to complete. Substantial tissue remodeling occurs during the ovulation, the follicle increases its own size, and the layers of theca cells fuse with the tunica albuginea, resulting into thinner and permitting rupturing of follicle to release the oocyte [4]. The mature oocyte when released by the rupturing of follicle its uptake facilitated by the fingure like opening projections of fallopian tube which is known as fimbriae, if fertilization occur here then the blastocyst further transfer it towards the uterus where the pregnancy takes place [5].

Inflammation is defensive mechanism of the cells that is crucial to health and it is delineated as a local immune response of living vascularized tissues to endogenous and exogenous stimuli and its actions is to removal of injurious stimuli with starting the healing process [6]. Inflammation is also initiated when the cells die from deficiency of nutrients or hypoxia, a condition that often is originated by the blood flow loss to the site. The chemical mediators of the inflammation generally originate from the blood plasma, platelets, white blood cells (monocytes, neutrophils, basophils, and macrophages), endothelial cells lining of the blood vessels, mast cells, and injured tissue cells. The chemical mediators responsible for the inflammation is histamine, that stimulates vasodilation and increases the vascular permeability, and lysosomal substances acting as vascular permeability enhancer which are secreted from neutrophils, and certain small proteins in the complement system, namely C3a and C5a. Various cytokines released by inflammatory cells also have vasoactive and chemotactic function. Many cells produce prostaglandins which linked to the fever and pain of inflammation; a group of fatty acids which involves in the augmentation of vascular permeability of the other substances, platelets aggregation; which is essential for coagulation [6].

The objective of this review is to understand and establish a relationship between how the inflammation as well as different mediators of inflammation that influence the ovulation process that is crucial for clinical management and prediction of gynecological complications for future study.

2. Inflammatory genetic mechanism

Inflammation is detected throughout many normal reproductive progressions, for the duration of ovulation, menstruation, implantation, as well as parturition. Ovulatory cycle is also considered as inflammatory process because the rupturing of dominant follicle undergoes the process of healing [7]. Throughout ovulation, the role of inflammation is very significant in terms of folliculogenesis and luteinization. In the course of the rupturing of follicle, there is significant surge of intra-follicular pressure which leads to weakening of follicle layer by the stimulation of gonadotropins resulted in inflammation [8]. The inflammation notably persuades in both ovulation and tissue remodeling phase which resulted in events of hyperemia, vasodilation, edema, collagenolysis, and proliferation of cells [1].

Wissing et al. isolated differentially expressed 1186 genes in human granulosa cells (GC) before and 36 h after the administration of hCG, besides 572 genes found to be up-regulated which represented angiogenesis, inflammation, extracellular matrix and growth factors and 614 genes down-regulated which denoted cell cycle and about 72 genes which has been earlier establish linked with ovarian cancer. H19/mir675, CD24, CLDN11, ANKRD22, and FBXO32 adds as new ovulation related genes and PTGS2, an inflammatory gene heavily up-regulated [5].

3. Inflammatory oxygen species and ovulation

The release of mature oocyte relies on the expansion of cumulus oocyte complex (COC), where the reactive oxygen species (ROS) function as critical modulator of inflammatory reaction. Residual growing follicles promoted to apoptosis by the ROS [8]. Simultaneously estrogen synthesis started with the influx of catalase and Glutathione (GSH) i.e. a non-enzymatic antioxidant species exists in oocytes and embryos, in growing residual follicles for the maintenance of normal ovarian function and counter the apoptotic process. The luteal phase begins with progesterone production for the maintenance of preliminary stage of pregnancy, if fertilization did not occur then degeneration of corpus luteum starts [2]. For the induction of cell proliferation, maturation, cellular-differentiation and ovulation the physiological level of ROS is very important [9]. Augmented ROS may outcomes to DNA damage, activation of signaling cascades, and epigenetic alterations [10]. Inflammation in the course of ovulation is also responsible for the oxidative stress, damaging of DNA and moreover in the neoplastic ovarian surface epithelium (OSE) cells transformation [11].

4. PCOS and inflammation

Elevated level of inflammation also involves in the pathogenicity of many reproductive disorder such as polycystic ovary syndrome (PCOS), characterized by biochemical hyperandrogenemia, chronic anovulation, and polycystic ovaries. About 5 to 15% of reproductive age woman are suffering with this disorder in the world. It is anticipated that the metabolic disorders associated with PCOS and the pathogenesis of PCOS due to systemic inflammation as well as dysfunctioning of mitochondria. About 33% adolescent PCOS girls are more prone to metabolic disorder are obese, which is 3 to 5 folds higher if compared with same age healthy girls and body mass index (BMI) [9]. Studies reported and found the significant increased level of monocytes, lymphocytes, CRP, interleukins IL-1, IL-6, IL-18, pro-inflammatory cytokines and TNF- α in addition to increased production of advanced oxidation protein, protein carbonylation and lipid peroxidation in PCOS patients compared with same reproductive aged healthy persons [9]. The PCOS patients suffered with chronic inflammation [12, 13]. Along with the deficiency of antioxidant i.e. Vitamin C, Vitamin E and Superoxide dismutases (SOD), this leads to cause inflammatory milieu and risk to develop the obesity, type-1 diabetes, insulin resistance, hyperandrogenism, and cardiovascular ailment [1, 14].

5. Anti-inflammatory agents and ovulation

The surge of luteinizing hormone (LH) stimulate the production of cyclic adenosine monophosphate (cAMP), steroidal hormones, histamine discharge and various mediators of inflammation e.g. prostaglandins, bradykinins, C-reactive protein (CRP), Proinflammatory cytokines, etc. [1]. Christina et al. study states that the successful folliculogenesis, oocyte maturation, and ovulation require a healthy inflammatory response.

There are many findings illustrate that the importance of untroubled inflammatory response for proper folliculogenesis and ovulation, if it altered, may contribute to oocyte quality concern and reproductive dysfunctions such as anovulation, infertility, menstrual irregularities, etc. [5, 8]. It is reported that low dose of Aspirin taken by the patients suffering with higher systemic inflammation were able to reestablish the pregnancy [4, 12].

6. Correlation between hormone and inflammation

The level of LH also positive correlation with release of prostaglandins and eicosanoids that are the source to trigger the fibroblasts, promotes the angiogenesis and hyperemia, collagenase activation, release of proteolytic enzymes, some of which degrade the follicular connective tissue resulting ovulation, and cause the inflammation. The gene hyaluronan (HA) synthase-2 (Has2) associated with COC matrix formation. Bradykinin play a key role in vasodilation which appears to be 10 folds increased during ovulation. The serum C- reactive protein (CRP), a marker of inflammation also raised to stimulate the production of interlukin-6 from macrophages, tumor necrosis factor α (TNFα) and the competent system of inflammatory response further activated by the adipocytes [13].

7. Role of proinflammatory cytokines

The role of proinflammatory cytokines is also important throughout folliculogenesis and induction of ovulation [5]. Higher level of follicular TNF-α resulted in the poor quality of oocyte which compromised with the fertility, also the elevated level of interleukin (IL-6) associated with less chances of conceiving while the another interleukin (IL-1) found to be regulated by FSH and its higher follicular level has been resulted in the higher chance on embryo implantation [7, 15].

8. Nucleotide leukin rich polypeptide -3 inflammasomes

A recent finding added a new mechanism for ovulatory process regulation, suggested that the NLRP3 activation of nucleotide leukin rich polypeptide 3 (NLRP3) inflammasomes started before the ovulation lasting completion of ovulation. They induces the follicular development by 52 hours' treatment using Pregnant mare serum gonadotropin (PMSG). It was found that the expression of NLRP3 inflammasomes and adaptor protein apoptosis-associated speck-like protein (ASC) significantly increased, and it was appeared a dramatic surge in caspase-1 activity and production of IL-1β [16].

9. Gonadotropin in inflammation

Gonadotropin surge trigger the ovlation with the parllel stimulation of two gens of preovulatory follicles in granulosa cells, prostaglandin-endoperoxide synthase 2 (PTGS2) and progesterone receptor (PGR). Secretion of LH stimulates the induction of both PTGS2 and PGR in preovulatory granulosa cells. Expression of PTGS2 stimulates inflammation by releasing pro-inflammatory prostaglandins wheras anti-inflammatory action through the PGR by the supression of pro-inflamatory genes or thru the stimulation of antiinflammatory genes. Higher level of PGE2 and PTGS2 are associated with the ovarian disorders such as ovarian carcinoma, ovarian hyperstimulation syndrome (OHSS) as well as polycystic ovarian syndrome (PCOS) [11].

10. Inflammatory prostaglandins

Prostaglandins (PGs) are signaling molecules derived from dietary fats with clinically relevant roles in reproductive biology. PGE2, for instance, promotes ovulation downstream of the luteinizing hormone surge. Excess consumption of nonsteroidal anti-inflammatory drugs, which inhibit prostaglandin-endoperoxide synthase (cyclooxygenase or Cox), is associated with reversible female infertility, likely due to failed ovulation. On the other hand, proinflammatory cytokines increase PGF2α associated with corpus luteum development and immune cell recruitment [17].

11. Adipokines

A study (Bongrani et, al.) based on the adipokines roles in the pathophysiology of PCOS, they analyzed the adipokines profile in the normal-weight PCOS patients and obese women with PCOS and comparison of these with the women whose only have a Polycystic ovary morphology. Whereas they found the PCOS patient reported with lower adiponectin level in serum as well as FF, and also the lower expression in adipose tissue of AdipoR1 and AdipoR2. In granulosa cells AdipoR1 expression was positively correlated with the follicular numbers, oocytes count and embryos, on the other hand there was no significant difference in AdipoR2 reporters was found. No correlation was established among the FF adiponectin concentration and expression of its receptor, AdipoR1/AdipoR2 in GCs. Dysregulation of adiponectin may be likely mechanisms which could be responsible for impairment of insulin-sensitivity in PCOS patient, and it seems to be independent of insulin resistance severity and a potential role of adiponectin in folliculogenesis.

12. Omentin

The concentration of Omentin in FF was found to be positively correlated with BMI, higher in obese patients compared to the normal weight patients. They also point out that the omentin may possibly be controlled by means of inflammation, because the expression of omentin altered in inflammatory conditions [18].

13. Oxidative stress

ROS is necessary to maintain the normal female reproductive physiology, it is involved in the oocyte maturation, corpus luteum apoptosis as well as embryonic development process. The release of mature oocyte depends on the expansion of cumulus oocyte complex (COC), where the reactive oxygen species (ROS) function as critical modulator of inflammatory reaction. The exposure of ROS may lead to undergo transformative alterations of epithelial cells in the ovary and fallopian tubes [10].

14. Tumor necrosis factor-α

It has a significant role in the process of ovulation as well as to excrete out the damaged corpous luteum from the ovarian tissue. It works by the ligand gated receptors, TNFR-I and TNFR-II [10, 19]. It is also linked with the various pathological conditions when its level elevated. It is also reported that the infertile women with PCOS reported to have higher free fatty acids and blood serum level of TNF-α when compared with the healthy patients. Oxidative stressed cells also found to release higher levels of TNF-α than the normal ovarian epithelial cells which results in an autocrine surge of TNF-α mRNA as well as in the form of expression in other pro-inflammatory cytokines, chemokines, and angiogenic factors [10, 20, 21].

15. Interleukins

Interleukin-15 is an important interleukin which is negatively associated with the oocyte maturation. It belongs to the cytokines family having four α-helix bundle, i.e. pleiotropic glycoprotein. It was reported to be higher in women with an unsuccessful assisted reproductive techniques outcomes (median value 1.4 pg./ml) than of the women those succeeded the clinical pregnancy (median value 0.8 pg./ml) [22]. The IL-6 is a regulator of cumulus cell-oocyte complex (COC) expansion and responsible for the quality of murine oocyte during the in-vitro fertilization.

16. Matrix metalloproteinases

The another factor which has been found to be involved in follicular development as well as in the ovulation process are Matrix metalloproteinases (MMPs). The matrix metalloproteinases activities regulated by the specific tissue inhibitors called metalloproteinases (TIMPs) and endogenous inhibitors. The balance of both these is very essential for their activity and to maintain the normal ovarian physiology. It is well noticed that the MMP-2 and MMP-9 level increased during and before the 3 hours of ovulation if compared to 20–22 hour before the ovulation. Augmented level of MMP-9 also postulated in the PCOS pathophysiology and is also linked with progression and etiological to many other ailments such as cystic fibrosis, asthma, ulcerative colitis, cardiovascular disorders, atherosclerosis, etc. [23, 24].

17. Peroxisome proliferator-activated receptor gamma

The Peroxisome Proliferator-Activated Receptor Gamma (PPAR-γ) is established to have an ability to prevent the expression of various signaling molecules also regulates the levels of prostaglandins through regulation of cyclooxygenase-2 and differentiation of immune cells especially those which are a part of inflammation. Thereby controls ovarian function, fertilization, and ovulation. Its proinflammatory activity is linked to the formation of prostaglandin E by downregulation of COX-2 mRNA of granulosa cells whereas it is upregulated twice in PCOS [25]. It is also being proven that the PPAR-γ controls genes responsible for expression of TNF-alpha and Interleukins along with others. The study is supported by use of PPAR-γ agonist which affected the functioning of ovaries by involving signal transduction of insulin and IGF [20].

18. Chemokines

Earlier study reported the expression of chemokine receptor-2 (C-C motif) (CCR2) in the human ovarian cumulus-oocyte complexes, theca cells, preovulatory follicles and in feline ovarian follicle walls. This receptor is believed to be involved in folliculogenesis and determines the reproductive lifespan of female [25] (**Figure 1**).

19. Conclusions

Inflammation is believed to be involved in triggering the process of ovulation. There are several factors, genes, receptors, proinflammatory mediators playing important but diverse role in ovulation. The extent of their role and intensity of reaction induced by them required to be studied to understand their clinical applicability.

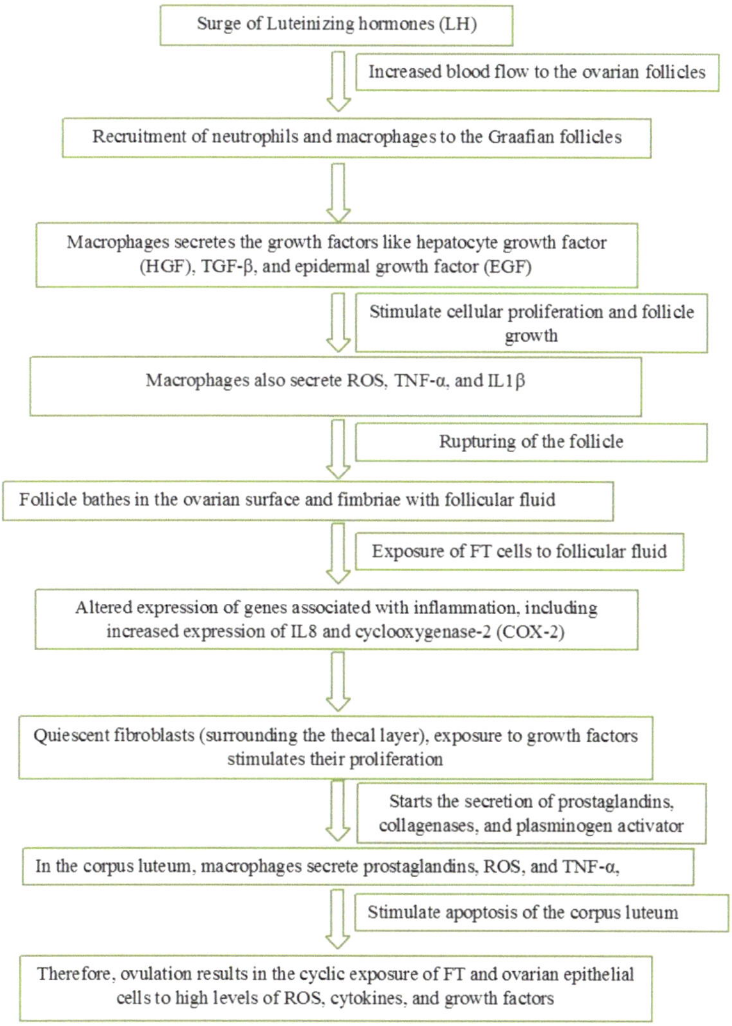

Figure 1.
Inflammatory process in ovulation.

Acknowledgements

We acknowledge the financial help received from Grant4Target.

Conflict of interest

The authors declare no conflict of interest.

Author details

Pankaj Pant and Havagiray R. Chitme*
Faculty of Pharmacy, DIT University, Dehradun, Uttarakhand, India

*Address all correspondence to: hrchitme@gmail.com

References

[1] Boots, C. E., & Jungheim, E. S. Inflammation and human ovarian follicular dynamics. In Seminars in reproductive medicine. 2015;33: 270.

[2] Mancini, V., & Pensabene, V. . Organs-On-Chip Models of the Female Reproductive System. Bioengineering. 2019; 6(4), 103.

[3] Souček, K., Malenovská, A., Kahounová, Z., Remšík, J., Holubcová, Z., Soukup, T., & Hampl, A.. Presence of growth/differentiation factor-15 cytokine in human follicular fluid, granulosa cells, and oocytes. Journal of assisted reproduction and genetics. 2018; 35(8), 1407-1417.

[4] Espey, L. L.. Comprehensive analysis of ovarian gene expression during ovulation using differential display. In Differential Display Methods and Protocols. Humana Press. 2006;219-241.

[5] Wissing, M. L., Kristensen, S. G., Andersen, C. Y., Mikkelsen, A. L., Høst, T., Borup, R., & Grøndahl, M. L.. Identification of new ovulation-related genes in humans by comparing the transcriptome of granulosa cells before and after ovulation triggering in the same controlled ovarian stimulation cycle. Human reproduction. 2014;29(5):997-1010.

[6] Agita, A., & Alsagaff, M. T.. Inflammation, immunity, and hypertension. Acta Med Indones. 2017;49(2):158-165.

[7] Papler, T. B., Bokal, E. V., Maver, A., Kopitar, A. N., & Lovrečić, L.. Transcriptomic analysis and meta-analysis of human granulosa and cumulus cells. PloS one. 2015;10(8):e0136473.

[8] Adams, J., Liu, Z., Ren, Y. A., Wun, W. S., Zhou, W., Kenigsberg, S., & Richards, J.. Enhanced inflammatory transcriptome in the granulosa cells of women with polycystic ovarian syndrome. The Journal of Clinical Endocrinology & Metabolism. 2016;101(9):3459-3468.

[9] Khashchenko, E., Vysokikh, M., Uvarova, E., Krechetova, L., Vtorushina, V., Ivanets, T., & Sukhikh, G.. Activation of Systemic Inflammation and Oxidative Stress in Adolescent Girls with Polycystic Ovary Syndrome in Combination with Metabolic Disorders and Excessive Body Weight. Journal of Clinical Medicine. 2020;9(5):1399.

[10] Savant, S. S., Sriramkumar, S., & O'Hagan, H. M.. The role of inflammation and inflammatory mediators in the development, progression, metastasis, and chemoresistance of epithelial ovarian cancer. Cancers. 2018;10(8):251.

[11] Park, C. J., Lin, P. C., Zhou, S., Barakat, R., Bashir, S. T., Choi, J. M., ... & Ko, C. J.. Progesterone Receptor Serves the Ovary as a Trigger of Ovulation and a Terminator of Inflammation. Cell reports. 2020;31(2): 107496.

[12] Radin, R. G., Sjaarda, L. A., Silver, R. M., Nobles, C. J., Mumford, S. L., Perkins, N. J., & Schisterman, E. F.. C-Reactive protein in relation to fecundability and anovulation among eumenorrheic women. Fertility and sterility. 2018;109(2):232-239.

[13] Shaaban, Z., Khoradmehr, A., Amiri-Yekta, A., Shirazi, M. R. J., & Tamadon, A.. Pathophysiologic mechanisms of obesity-and chronic inflammation-related genes in etiology of polycystic ovary syndrome. Iranian Journal of Basic Medical Sciences. 2019;22(12):1378.

[14] Wang, S., He, G., Chen, M., Zuo, T., Xu, W., & Liu, X.. The

role of antioxidant enzymes in the ovaries. Oxidative medicine and cellular longevity. 2017;2017. DOI: 10.1155/2017/4371714

[15] Da Broi, M. G., Giorgi, V. S. I., Wang, F., Keefe, D. L., Albertini, D., & Navarro, P. A.. Influence of follicular fluid and cumulus cells on oocyte quality: clinical implications. Journal of assisted reproduction and genetics. 2018;35(5):735-751.

[16] Zhang, Z., Wang, F., & Zhang, Y.. Expression and contribution of nlrp3 inflammasome during the follicular development induced by PMSG. Frontiers in Cell and Developmental Biology. 2019;7:256.

[17] Pier, B., Edmonds, J. W., Wilson, L., Arabshahi, A., Moore, R., Bates, G. W., & Miller, M. A.. Comprehensive profiling of prostaglandins in human ovarian follicular fluid using mass spectrometry. Prostaglandins & other lipid mediators. 2018;134:7-15.

[18] Bongrani, A., Mellouk, N., Rame, C., Cornuau, M., Guérif, F., Froment, P., & Dupont, J.. Ovarian Expression of Adipokines in Polycystic Ovary Syndrome: A Role for Chemerin, Omentin, and Apelin in Follicular Growth Arrest and Ovulatory Dysfunction?. International journal of molecular sciences. 2019;20(15):3778.

[19] Gupta, M., Babic, A., Beck, A. H., & Terry, K.. TNF-α expression, risk factors, and inflammatory exposures in ovarian cancer: evidence for an inflammatory pathway of ovarian carcinogenesis?. Human pathology. 2016;54:82-91.

[20] Lee, J. Y., Tae, J. C., Kim, C. H., Hwang, D., Kim, K. C., Suh, C. S., & Kim, S. H.. Expression of the genes for peroxisome proliferator-activated receptor-γ, cyclooxygenase-2, and proinflammatory cytokines in granulosa cells from women with polycystic ovary syndrome. Clinical and experimental reproductive medicine. 2017;44(3):146.

[21] Kowsar, R., Keshtegar, B., & Miyamoto, A.. Understanding the hidden relations between pro-and anti-inflammatory cytokine genes in bovine oviduct epithelium using a multilayer response surface method. Scientific reports. 2019;9(1):1-17.

[22] Spanou, S., Kalogiannis, D., Zapanti, E., Gazouli, M., Sfontouris, I. A., Siristatidis, C., & Mastorakos, G.. Interleukin 15 concentrations in follicular fluid and their effect on oocyte maturation in subfertile women undergoing intracytoplasmic sperm injection. Journal of assisted reproduction and genetics. 2018;35(6):1019-1025.

[23] Daan, N. M., Koster, M. P., de Wilde, M. A., Dalmeijer, G. W., Evelein, A. M., Fauser, B. C., & de Jager, W.. Biomarker profiles in women with PCOS and PCOS offspring; a pilot study. PLoS One. 2016;11(11):e0165033.

[24] Hrabia, A., Wolak, D., Kwaśniewska, M., Kieronska, A., Socha, J. K., & Sechman, A.. Expression of gelatinases (MMP-2 and MMP-9) and tissue inhibitors of metalloproteinases (TIMP-2 and TIMP-3) in the chicken ovary in relation to follicle development and atresia. Theriogenology. 2019;125,268-276.

[25] Santos, A. G. A., Pereira, L. A. A. C., Viana, J. H. M., Russo, R. C., & Campos-Junior, P. H. A.. The CC-chemokine receptor 2 is involved in the control of ovarian folliculogenesis and fertility lifespan in mice. Journal of Reproductive Immunology. 2020;141:103174.

Section 2

Diagnosis

Chapter 3

Extra-Uterine Fibroids

Rakesh Kumar Gupta and Poonam Wasnik

Abstract

Leiomyomas are the most common gynecologic and uterine neoplasms. Uterine leiomyomas present in approximately 25% of women during reproductive age. Extrauterine leiomyomas (EULs) are rarer and usually arise in the genitourinary tract, however, may arise at nearly any anatomic location and possess a great diagnostic challenge. Moreover, the EULs may also present with unusual growth patterns such as disseminated peritoneal leiomyomatosis, intravenous leiomyomatosis, benign metastasizing leiomyoma, parasitic leiomyoma, and retroperitoneal mass. However, the cell of origin from smooth muscle cells and histological benign characteristics is similar to their uterine counterpart. The presence of a synchronous uterine leiomyoma or history of previous hysterectomy is a considerable evidence for the diagnosis of these abnormally located and unusual growth pattern displaying EULs. Different imaging modalities like ultrasonography, computed tomography, and magnetic resonance imaging are helpful in the diagnosis of EULs, however, sometimes a histopathological examination is required for the confirmation.

Keywords: Extrauterine, leiomyoma, disseminated peritoneal leiomyomatosis, benign metastasizing leiomyoma, parasitic leiomyoma, genitourinary tract

1. Introduction

Leiomyomas are benign smooth muscle tumours usually arise from the uterus [1]. Classical uterine leiomyoma manifest as firm, well circumscribed mass, and localized to the pelvic cavity [2]. Extrauterine leiomyomas (EULs) are very rare and their etiology is not clear [1]. They grow in unusual patterns and locations, thus possess greater diagnostic challenge. Different presentations of EUL are disseminated peritoneal leiomyomatosis (DPL), parasitic leiomyoma (PL), uterine-like mass lesions, adenomyoma and endomyometriosis [3]. Unusual sites involvement like vulval and rectovaginal leiomyomas are also found [4]. EULs arising in the gastrointestinal tract, genitourinary tract, as well as other rare locations including sinonasal cavities, orbits, and skin are also described in some case reports.

Uterine leiomyoma is a benign tumour which originates from smooth muscle cells. Leiomyomas can present in abnormal growth patterns and tend to occur in extrauterine location especially in cases with prior history of hysterectomy or surgery for uterine leiomyomas.

2. Types of EULs

2.1 Disseminated peritoneal leiomyomatosis

Multifocal proliferation of multiple smooth nodules throughout the peritoneal surface histologically similar to uterine myomas is known as leiomyomatosis peritonealis disseminate (LPD) or disseminated peritoneal leiomyomatosis (DPL) [3, 5, 6]. The peritoneal cavity shows multiple nodules of smooth muscle (**Figure 1**) [6, 7]. DPL usually occurs in reproductive age group with an indolent course, and are mostly detected incidentally [6]. Uterine myoma morcellation is a known risk factor for the development of DPL with an incidence rate around 0.12 to 0.95% after morcellation [5, 6]. Morcellation may lead to spreading of cellular materials of the myoma fragments. These morcellated tissues get disseminated if they are not removed and may become infarcted, necrotic or even parasitic [3]. Other causes which can contribute in the pathogenesis of DPL includes; hormonal, genetic, and sub-peritoneal mesenchymal stem cells metaplasia.

Pelvic region is the commonest site especially in pouch of douglas, may also spread to entire abdomen to involve omentum and mesentery. DPL is very invasive and very difficult for complete surgical excision, which may invade into bladder, retroperitoneal space, liver and small bowel [5]. They present as numerous subcentimetric grey -white firm nodules, sometimes with solid cystic hemorrhagic changes [5]. DPL can presents with ascites and adenopathy, which can be confused with peritoneal carcinomatosis. Sometimes, DPL may evolve into leiomyosarcoma, though it is extremely rare and possess high mortality rate [5, 6]. Due to unusual multifocal presentation, peritoneal myomas mimic malignant peritoneal tumor, so aggressive treatment at first surgical line should be avoided [6].

Some cases of gastrointestinal tract (GIT) leiomyomas have been reported with intestinal obstruction or bleeding without past or present history of uterine fibroid. But GIT leiomyomas are different from LPD. GIT leiomyomas can develop from intestinal wall and may reach the lumen whereas LPD mostly reach peritoneal cavity and omentum [5]. But disseminated GIT leiomyoma could be related to LPD, if there is no evidence of uterine myomas [5].

2.2 Benign metastasizing leiomyoma

Benign metastasizing leiomyoma (BML) is a rare condition that affects women with a history of uterine myomectomy, which is found to metastasize to extra-uterine sites. The disease is characterized by monoclonal proliferation of smooth muscle cells and haematogenous spread from uterine leiomyoma to distant locations, most commonly

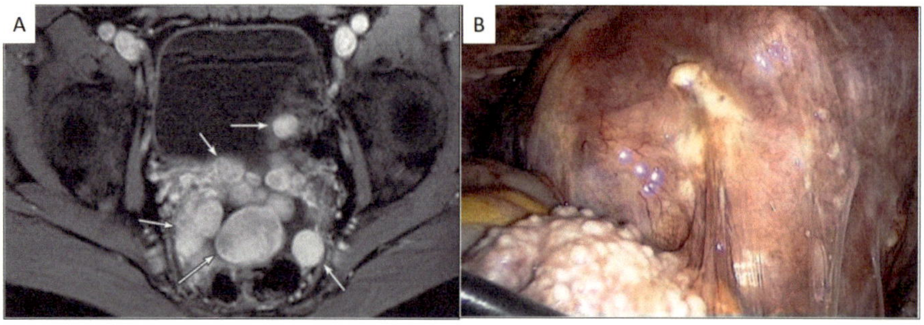

Figure 1.
(A) Contrast-enhanced T1-weighted fat-suppressed fast spin echo magnetic resonance image shows multiple homogeneously enhancing peritoneal leiomyomas (arrows), (B) Intra-operative gross image showing multiple variably sized peritoneal nodules representing disseminated peritoneal leiomyomatosis.

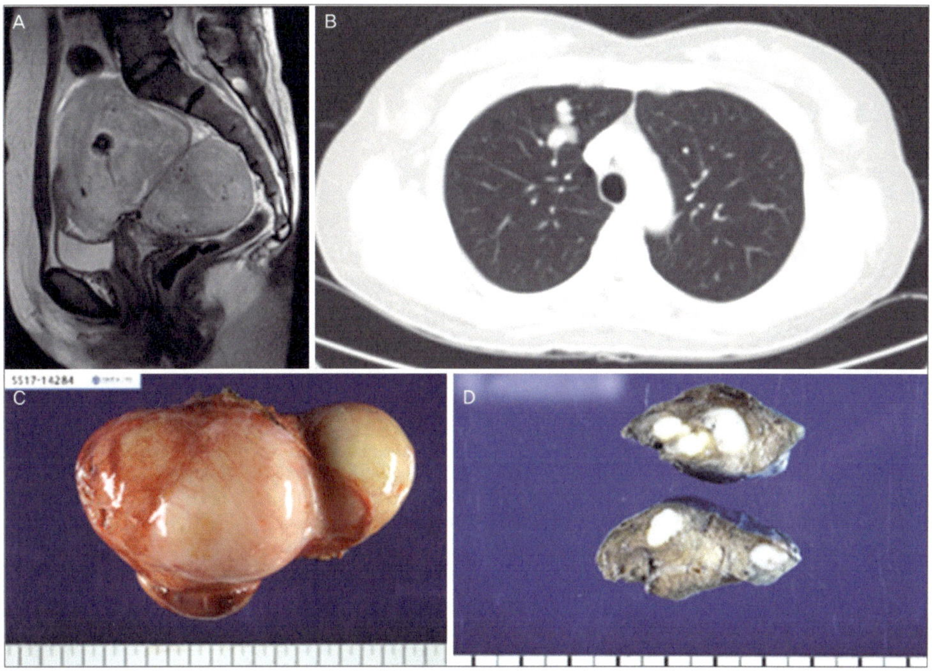

Figure 2.
(A) Abdomino-pelvic computed tomography showing a large pelvic mass, and (B) thoracic computed tomography showing bilateral lung nodules, Gross specimens (C) pelvic mass excision and (D) video-assisted thoracoscopic guided surgical resection of bilateral basal lung nodule in an operated case of total abdominal hysterectomy with bilateral salpingo-oopherectomy.

the lungs (**Figure 2**) [2, 8]. The other uncommon site of metastasis includes heart and spinal cord [2]. Metaplastic transformation of the coelomic epithelium may explain BML in almost any place where mesothelial mesenchyme exists [2]. BML commonly occur during peri-menopausal period. Surgical excision is the treatment of choice.

2.3 Intravenous leiomyomatosis

Intravenous leiomyomatosis (IVL) also included under smooth muscle tumours with unusual growth pattern like that of benign metastasizing leiomyoma (BML) and diffuse peritoneal leiomyomatosis (DPL) and difficult to distinguish from them [2]. IVL is very rare variant of benign leiomyomas. It presents as fragile and malleable leiomyoma that extends through adjacent venous structures in a worm-like fashion (**Figure 3**) [2]. Rarey, IVL may infiltrate into the right heart chamber and the lungs [6]. Due to wide range of clinical manifestation, IVL is difficult to diagnose pre-operatively [2].

2.4 Parasitic leiomyoma

Parasitic leiomyoma is termed when leiomyoma especially subserous fibroid is pedunculated off the uterine serosa or when fragments of a fibroid detach, get implanted and grow within the peritoneal cavity or becomes adherent to other structures, especially the omentum (**Figure 4**) [3]. They obtain their blood supply from nearby organ and the uterine pedicle either or become avascular and disappear completely. These are also known as ectopic leiomyoma [3]. Cucinella et al. suggested morcellated hysterectomies or myomectomies as an important cause for development of parasitic leiomyoma [9].

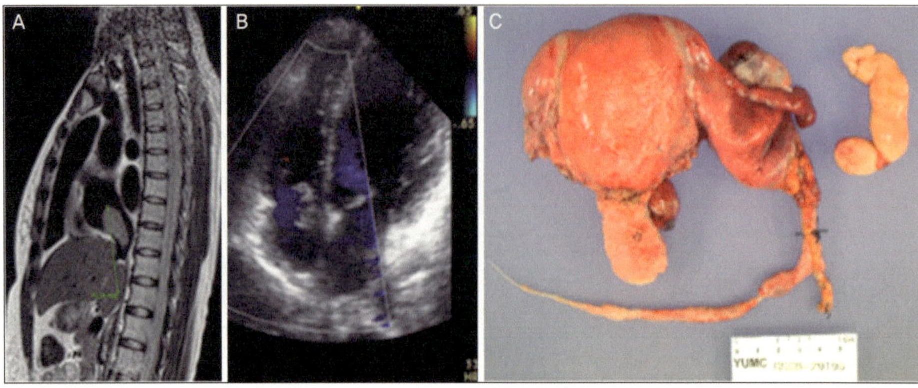

Figure 3.
(A) Magnetic resonance image showing a 'comma' shaped thrombosis, extending from the intrahepatic portion of inferior vena cava (IVC) to the right atrium, (B) Echocardiography showing an intracardiac mass with dynamic movement past the tricuspid valve into the right ventricle, (C) Gross specimen of total abdominal hysterectomy with left salpingo-oophorectomy, and IVC and intracardiac mass.

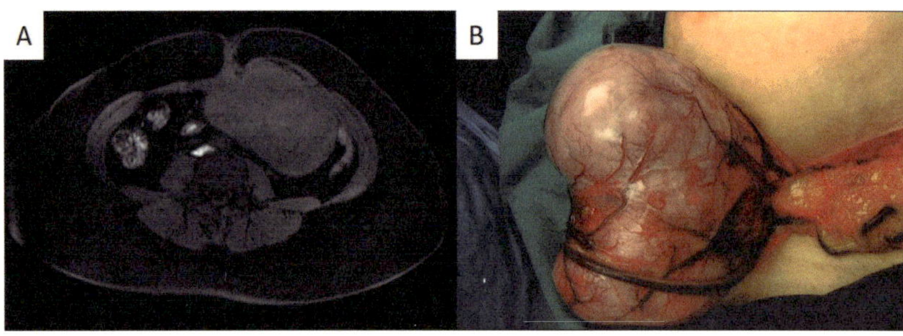

Figure 4.
(A) Magnetic resonance image showing two large lobulated peritoneal masses with similar signal and enhancement characteristics, (B) Gross specimen of peritoneal fibroid vascularized by omental vessels in a patient underwent laparoscopic myomectomy 5 years earlier.

2.5 Extrauterine adenomyoma

Extrauterine adenomyomas (EUA) are benign tumours composed of smooth muscles, endometrial glands and endometrial stroma (**Figure 5**) [10]. In the literature, four hypotheses have been proposed for the development of EUA which includes (1) Müllerian duct fusion defect - the failure of fusion of Müllerian ducts result in either duplication or atresia of the uterus which is suggested by the formation of uterine-like masses, (2) Subcoelomic mesenchyme transformation - Subcoelomic mesenchyme is a layer of tissue that lies underneath the mesothelial surface of the peritoneum. It also lies underneath the subserosal stroma of uterus, uterine ligaments, ovaries and fallopian tubes, (3) Müllerianosis - It is a heterotopic Müllerian rests incorporated into other organs during organogenesis which may proliferate in response to hormones and (4) Endomyometriosis - along with endomyometriosis, smooth muscle hyperplasia or metaplasia leads to EUA [11, 12].

3. Role of hormones

Leiomyomas are clonal neoplasm and express more number of estrogen and progesterone receptors in comparison to normal myometrium [1, 2]. Circulating estrogen, progesterone and other growth factors like epidermal growth factor and

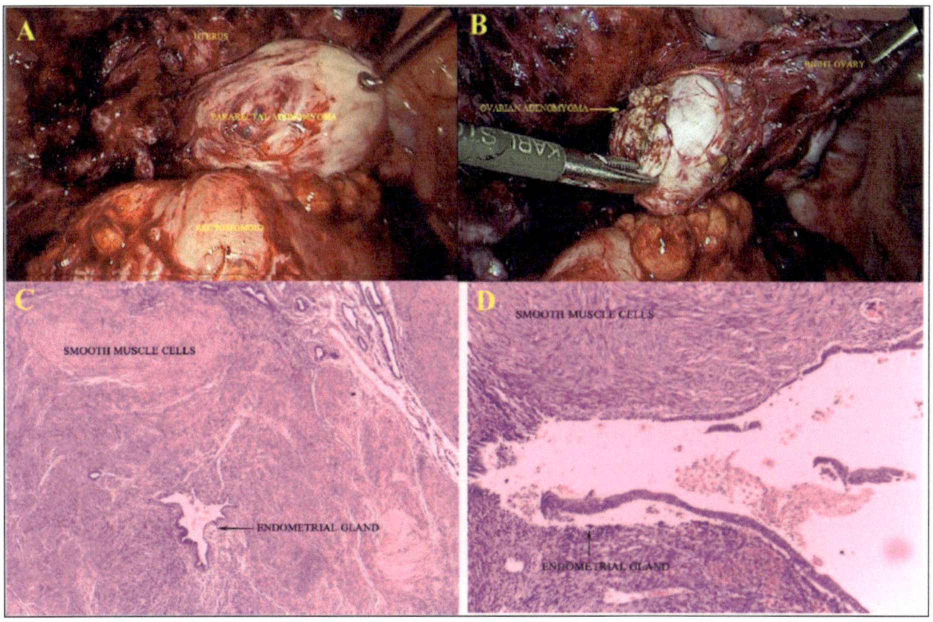

Figure 5.
Intra-operative laparoscopic images of (A) pararectal adenomyoma and (B) right ovarian adenomyoma, histopathology images of ovarian adenomyoma (C) low power and (D) high power delineating smooth muscle bundles with embedded endometrial glands in a patient underwent laparoscopic myomectomy 5 years earlier.

insulin like growth factors are involved in the growth of uterine leiomyomas [1]. Estrogen stimulates the growth of leiomyoma independent of its location whether uterine or extrauterine [1]. However, the role of progesterone remains uncertain in extrauterine leiomyoma and it's serum levels are either normal or low. Withdrawal of progesterone and of sex steroid down regulates expression of estrogen receptors (ER) in both leiomyomas and myometrium. This indicates that progesterone and progestins have a dual role on leiomyomas. First, limitation of the tissue response due to blocking of ER replacement and leading to unopposed estrogenic growth effect either by direct stimulation or by increased expression of progesterone receptors (PR). Second, progesterone may leads to an intrinsic growth-stimulation [1]. Progesterone causes increased mitotic division causing myoma growth and leads to the higher propensity for development of the somatic mutations in the myomas. It is suggested that PR is highly expressed in leiomyomas occurring in the reproductive period [1]. Such hormones influence rapid increase in size of leiomyoma in pregnancy which may lead to fetal wastage. However, there is lower expression of PR in EUL than in UL suggesting that different factors may contribute to the development of these tumours. Sen et al found a significant difference for labeling indices of PR between UL and EUL, however it was not significant for ER. Thus, therapeutic models targeting PRs may not be effective on EUL.

4. Diagnosis

Patient may present with menorrhagia, or diagnosed incidentally with the history of previous myoma or myomectomy [3]. Ultrasound is useful for diagnosis of uterine fibroid. Prior diagnosis of extra-uterine fibroids is often difficult owing to non-specific clinical and radiological findings. MRI is very helpful when ultrasound shows poor delineation, and in case of rapidly growing fibroid suspicious for malignant transformation. MRI is also very useful for the diagnosis of DPL as well as to determine its extent of spread for surgical planning (**Figure 1A**) [3]. In case of IVL, apart from trans-vaginal ultrasound, and other modalities such as pelvic MRI, trans-thoracic echocardiography, abdomen or chest computed tomography (CT), and positron emission tomography (PET) are beneficial [2]. But there is limitation of MRI in locating retroperitoneal leiomyoma in which exact anatomical location can be often ascertained only intraoperatively [3]. Few cases may turn into leiomyosarcoma. Peritoneal cytology should be done in case of ascites [3].

Despite the extrauterine manifestation of leiomyoma, benign leiomyomas can be distinguished from leiomyosarcoma histologically. Sarcoma is marked by high grade cellular atypia, mitotic index of greater than 10, and presence of coagulative tumor cell necrosis [2]. IVL, usually found within uterine venous channels and microscopically shows benign appearing smooth muscle cells with low mitotic activity which stain for actin and desmin [2].

Recent investigations showed that IVL and BML share the same cytogenetic origin, demonstrated by comparative genomic hybridization, clonal number, and copy variance [2]. Leiomyoma and leiomyosarcoma both shows smooth muscle differentiation, however biologically they are different in relation to clinical, cytogenetic, and molecular features [13]. MED12, the mediator complex subunit 12 gene, is a recently described oncogene found in both primary and metastatic leiomyosarcoma. It is detected in as many as 70% of sporadic uterine leiomyoma [13]. Oncogenic roles of MED 12 gene is also detected in smooth muscle tumours arising in extrauterine locations, however, further validating studies required for confirming its exact role in their pathogenesis [13].

5. Treatment

Complete surgical excision is considered the mainstay and definitive treatment for EULs [14]. LPD mimics carcinomatosis, so total abdominal hysterectomy along with bilateral oophorectomy is often the preferred surgical treatment [5]. However, spontaneous regression has been also described in few case reports in the literature [5]. Surgical treatment affects reproductive ability in pre-menopausal women, so it should always be planned considering the family planning of the patient. In such situation diagnosis by intra-operative frozen section is very helpful [5]. Young patient in child bearing age group, especially who shows positivity for ER or PR markers in EUL, should be subject to ovary-sparing procedures and might be benefited from adjuvant therapy using GnRH agonist [2]. In histological proven DPL cases, debulking is very effective for relieving symptoms, provided the appropriate evaluation of general health conditions of the patient [5]. In unresectable cases of EULs, a medical treatment with aromatase inhibitors, chemotherapeutic agents or a gonadotropin agonist can be considered [2, 6]. During morcellation, falling pieces of myoma fragments should be avoided and proper attention should be given during removal via the port site. Post morcellation, reverse trendelenburg position should be attempted and thorough inspection with copious peritoneal lavage is recommended to aid the removal of remnant myoma pieces [3]. The Food and Drug Administration guidelines discourage the uses of laparoscopic power morcellation during hysterectomy or myomectomy for the treatment of uterine fibroids [3].

6. Follow-up

A routine follow-up is advised in all the patients of uterine fibroid undergoing morcellation for the development of EUL. Similarly, a long-term follow-up is essential in all the operated cases of EUL, particularly, DPL. In EULs, recurrence, if any, usually occur within 6 months after surgical resection. Since, these tumours are hormone sensitive, they usually show regression after reduction in estrogen exposure like after attainment of menopause. Repeat surgeries for recurrent EULs usually entail greater surgical difficulty and risks including visceral injuries [3].

7. Complications

DPL may leads to peritonitis and bowel obstruction which can result into sepsis and gangrene. Also, recurrence is not unusual in DPL cases due extensive involvement of peritoneal cavity. Sometimes, malignant transformation may occur in long standing cases.

8. Conclusions

EULs possess a great diagnostic challenge due to abnormal locations as well as their unusual growth patterns and more commonly associated with the complications in comparison to uterine leiomyomas. Though, histologically they show similarities with their uterine counter parts, however their pathogenesis is different and yet not well understood. These EULs, are hormone sensitive and may regress automatically after the recession of hormonal sources, however, this phenomenon is not universal in all cases. Due to their higher propensity for recurrence and rare malignant transformation a close follow-up is required. A peritoneal cytology and/or frozen section examination is recommended before major surgical procedures in EULs.

Source of financial support and conflict of interest

None to declare.

Declarations

Authors declare that all the necessary permissions has been obtained for using the images from the corresponding authors/editors of the concerned articles and all the papers from which these images reproduced has been cited.

Author details

Rakesh Kumar Gupta* and Poonam Wasnik
Department of Pathology and Laboratory Medicine, AIIMS, Raipur, C.G., India

*Address all correspondence to: rakesh.newjobi@gmail.com

References

[1] Sen N, Demirkan NC, Colakoglu N, Duzcan SE. Are there any differences in the expression of hormonal receptors and proliferation markers between uterine and extrauterine leiomyomas? International Journal of Surgical Pathology. 2008;**16**(1):43-47

[2] Kim YN, Eoh KJ, Lee JY, Nam EJ, Kim S, Kim SW, et al. Aberrant uterine leiomyomas with extrauterine manifestation: intravenous leiomyomatosis and benign metastasizing leiomyomas. Obstet Gynecol Sci. 2018;**61**(4):509-519

[3] Chin H, Ong XH, Yam PK, Chern BS. Extrauterine fibroids: a diagnostic challenge and a long-term battle. BMJ Case Rep. 2014;2014:bcr2014204928.

[4] Parry-Smith W. Extrauterine leiomyoma. Journal of Obstetrics and Gynaecology. 2010;**30**(3):317

[5] Gaichies L, Fabre-Monplaisir L, Fauvet R, Alves A, Mulliri A. Leiomyomatosis peritonealisis disseminata: Two unusual cases with literature review. J Gynecol Obstet Hum Reprod. 2018;**47**(2):89-94

[6] Tourlakis D, Tas B, Van Herendael B. Disseminated peritoneal leiomyomatosis. Gynecological Surgery. 2010;7:241-243

[7] Fasih N, Prasad Shanbhogue AK, Macdonald DB, Fraser-Hill MA, Papadatos D, Kielar AZ, et al. Leiomyomas beyond the uterus: unusual locations, rare manifestations. Radiographics. 2008;**28**(7):1931-1948

[8] Barnaś E, Książek M, Raś R, Skręt A, Skręt-Magierło J, Dmoch-Gajzlerska E. Benign metastasizing leiomyoma: A review of current literature in respect to the time and type of previous gynecological surgery. PLoS One. 2017;**12**(4):e0175875

[9] Cucinella G, Granese R, Calagna G, Somigliana E, Perino A. Parasitic myomas after laparoscopic surgery: an emerging complication in the use of morcellator? Description of four cases. Fertility and Sterility. 2011;**96**(2):e90-e96

[10] Paul PG, Gulati G, Shintre H, Mannur S, Paul G, Mehta S. Extrauterine adenomyoma: a review of the literature. European Journal of Obstetrics, Gynecology, and Reproductive Biology. 2018;**228**:130-136

[11] Moghadamfalahi M, Metzinger DS. Multiple extrauterine adenomyomas presenting in upper abdomen and pelvis: a case report and brief review of the literature. Case Reports in Obstetrics and Gynecology. 2012;**2012**:565901

[12] Huanwen W, Hui Z, Xiaowei X, Zhaohui L. Extrauterine adenomyoma of the liver with a focally cellular smooth muscle component occurring in a patient with a history of myomectomy: case report and review of the literature. Diagnostic Pathology. 2013;**8**:131

[13] Ravegnini G, Mariño-Enriquez A, Slater J, Eilers G, Wang Y, Zhu M, et al. MED12 mutations in leiomyosarcoma and extrauterine leiomyoma. Modern Pathology. 2013;**26**(5):743-749

[14] Sewell CA, Russo ML. Retroperitoneal leiomyoma: a case report. The Journal of Reproductive Medicine. 2011;**56**:515-517

Chapter 4

Fibroids and Hysteroscopy: An Overview

Cinta Vidal Mazo

Abstract

Submucosal fibroids account for 10% of total fibroids. They significantly impact quality of life causing abnormal uterine bleeding (AUB), reduction in fertility rates/infertility, obstetrics complications and abdominal pain. They are a major public health concern because of economic cost their monitoring and treatment requires. Hysteroscopic myomectomy is the first line minimally invasive and conservative surgical treatment. Treating a fibroid correctly implies knowing its physiopathology: What is a submucosal fibroids and what is its origin, what is the Pseudocapsule?. Proper diagnosis and standardized classification such as the Wamsteker classification are required. What are the limits to perform a hysteroscopic myomectomy? What devices are currently used? What are the requirements for conducting myomectomy procedures in the outpatient setting?. Different forms of surgical approach. Complications and consequences of a myomectomy. What will we do in the future with the management of small submucosal fibroids in asymptomatic patients with future genetic desires and can we resect type 3 fibroids by hysteroscopy avoiding a higher risk surgery by abdominal route?

Keywords: submucosal fibroid, pseudocapsule, hysteroscopic approach, outpatient myomectomy, economic impact

1. Introduction

Uterine fibroids are the most common benign pelvic tumors of the female genital tract. Their incidence is approximately 25–30% and may be higher depending on race, family history and genetics. Although most fibroid tumors are asymptomatic, they are a significant health issue due to the economic cost incurred by healthcare systems to monitor and treat them. The impact on the quality of life of women with this condition can be considerable.

Direct medical care expenses include surgery, treatment expenses for outpatient care and monitoring expenses. The indirect expenses include costs derived from inability to work and deterioration in the ability to perform usual tasks. Moreover, they include the expenses for obstetrical complications related to their presence or treatment. Obstetrical morbidity costs amount to $7.76 billion in the annual costs of myoma in the US. They cost more each year in the US than breast, ovarian and colon cancer [1–3].

When talking about fibroids and hysteroscopy, we are talking about submucosal fibroids, since they are the types of fibroids in the FIGO classification that can be approached in this way (FIGO Leiomyoma classification system) (**Figure 1**).

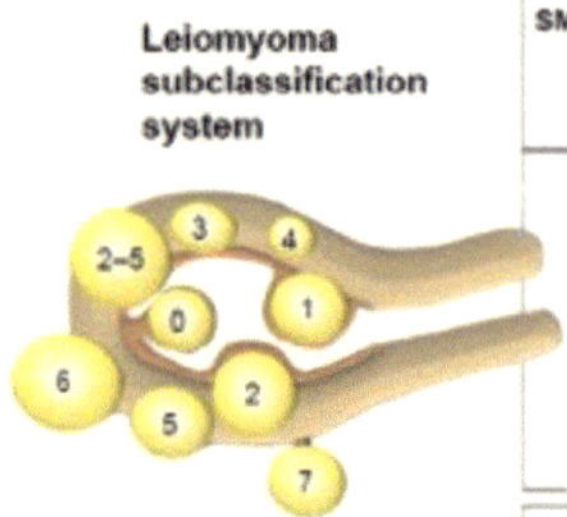

SM – Submucosal	0	Pedunculated intracavitary
	1	<50% intramural
	2	≥50% intramural
O – Other	3	Contacts endometrium; 100% intramural
	4	Intramural
	5	Subserosal ≥50% intramural
	6	Subserosal <50% intramural
	7	Subserosal pedunculated
	8	Other (specify eg. cervical, parasitic)
Hybrid leiomyomas (impact both endometrium and serosa)	Two numbers are listed separated by a hypen. By convention, the first refers to the relationship with the endometrium, while the second refers to the relationship to the serosa. One example is given below	
	2–5	Submucosal and subserosal, each with less than half the diameter in the endometerial and peritoneal cavities, respectively

Figure 1.
FIGO Leiomyomas subclassification system.

Submucosal fibroids amount to 5.5–10% of all uterine fibroids. They are frequently associated with abnormal uterine bleeding and infertility: women with submucous myomas are less likely to conceive, have significantly higher miscarriage rates and lower rates of successful deliveries, regardless of the conceptive method. There is scientific proof to support this fact. They have an impact on the functioning of the uterus and they cause changes in the normal anatomy of the uterus, alterations in blood supply, increased contractility, local hormonal changes and an action on the genetic expression of the endometrium (the endometrial RNA levels of HOXA11, LIF and BTEB1 decrease significantly in unfertile patients with uterine fibromas compared to healthy fertile control subjects at the moment of implantation). Removal of the myoma increases the fertility potential and the IVF results, increasing pregnancy rates from 17% to up to 80% according to the series. Therefore, it is reasonable to recommend surgical treatment in women who want to get pregnant and women that present abnormal uterine bleeding (AUB) [4–6].

Hysteroscopic myomectomy can be considered as the first-line minimally-invasive surgical treatment for submucosal myomas. This technique allows submucosal fibroids to be removed and the uterus to be preserved with minimal complications and rapid recovery times [7–10].

The execution of surgical hysteroscopy on an outpatient setting has turned into the gold standard of the medical practice.

There are many benefits to performing hysteroscopy in an outpatient setting, provided it is done safely and effectively, compared to hysteroscopy in the operating room: it does not require hospital admission, preoperative testing, or general or local anesthesia; it decreases post-surgical recovery times and overall procedure costs and it improves procedure satisfaction level for both healthcare providers and patients [11–15].

2. Submucosal myoma. Physiopathology

Submucosal fibroids are those fibroids that grow into the uterine cavity (**Figure 2**).

2.1 Origin submucosal fibroid

In order to treat a fibroid correctly, we must know its origin and the concept of pseudocapsule.

Fibroids are benign tumors that develop from a myometrial cell. It is not known why a myometrial cell starts multiplying uncontrollably, but we do know that their growth is estrogen-dependent. Fibroids have the mechanical capacity to push the healthy myometrium around them; the mechanical properties of fibroids are a key factor in their growth. Due to the compression exerted on surrounding structures, the fibroid induces gradual formation of a protective structure known as pseudocapsule that separates the fibroids from healthy uterine tissue. They grow inside the myometrium towards the least-resistance zone and, in the case of submucous myomas, they grow into the endometrial cavity. Submucosal myomas G0, G1 and G2 are classified as different transition phases of the same myoma [16] (**Figure 3**).

2.2 Pseudocapsule

Pseudocapsules are entities whose existence has been proven both histologically and through Doppler echography (this structure is seen as a ring of fire on an echogram). It has a different genetic expression profile than a normal myometrium and the surrounding myoma. This pseudocapsule is an independent entity, expressed as a layer between myometrium and myoma. It is comprised of collagen fibers,

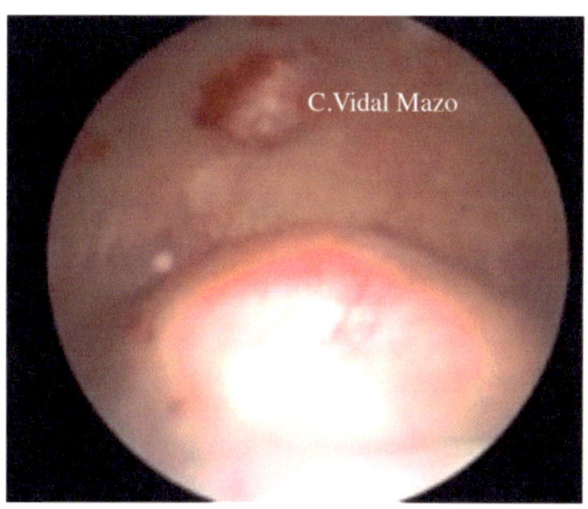

Figure 2.
Submucosal fibroid.

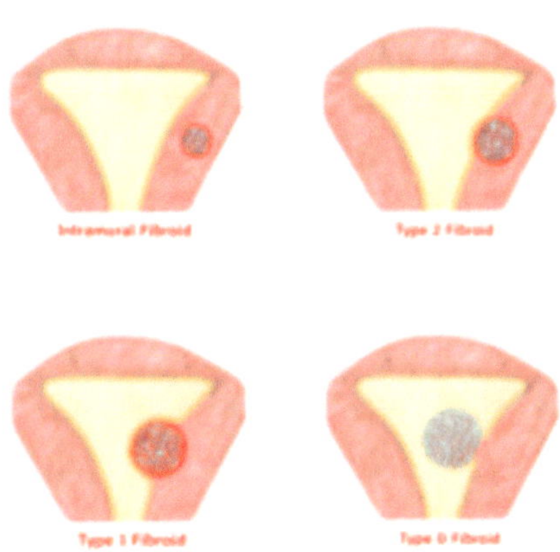

Figure 3.
Transition phases of fibroids.

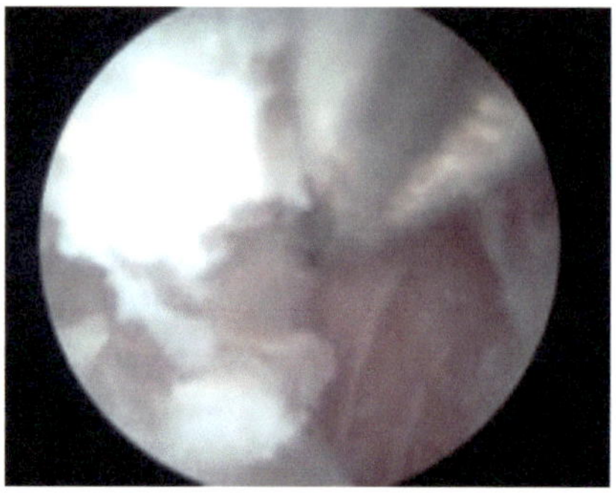

Figure 4.
Pseudocapsule and abscission plane.

blood vessels and neurofibers and it is rich in neuropeptides and neurotransmitters. These substances are believed to have an important role in wound healing and nerve repair, and they may be important for sexual and reproductive functions after resection of the myoma.

The fibroid is anchored through the pseudocapsule through connective bridges and small vessels creating a clear abscission plane between the fibroid and the pseudocapsule.

Contrary to popular belief, and except for pedunculated fibroids, other fibroids do not have a vascular pedicle that feeds them. The neurovascular network of the pseudocapsule is responsible for their irrigation (**Figure 4**) [17, 18].

3. Hysteroscopy: diagnosis and treatment

Hysteroscopy is currently the gold standard used to diagnose and determine the feasibility of resection of submucosal fibroids. It allows direct visualization of the uterine cavity and the identification of other intracavitary lesions. However, it only provides a subjective assessment of the size of the fibroid and indirect information about the degree of extension of the fibroid into the endometrial cavity.

3.1 Historical perspective

During the last two decades, thanks to advances in instruments and refinement of techniques, hysteroscopic myomectomy has acquired the status of 'surgical technique' and, today, represents the minimally invasive standard surgical procedure for the treatment of fibroids totally or mostly located in the uterine cavity.

William Norment performed the first hysteroscopic myomectomy in 1957 using the cutting handle. In 1976, Neuwirth and Amin reported a transcervical approach to excision of fibroids using a combination of techniques such as electrocautery and egg forceps. Neuwirth subsequently introduced a new technique for the resection of submucosal fibroids using the urologic resectoscope in 1978. Glycine (1.5% solution) was used for the first time by Haning et al. as a means of distention. Hallez created a specially designed dual-flow resectoscope for the uterus that allows full myomectomies even in cases of embedded fibroids. The gynecological resectoscope is currently the instrument of choice for the treatment of submucosal fibroids but mechanical morcellators are gaining popularity due to their mechanical characteristics for the performance of myomectomy and their lower rates of complications and synechiae after myoma surgery [19–23].

3.2 Other diagnostic procedures

There are other less invasive diagnostic procedures such as sonohysterography (SHG) that can provide better objective knowledge of the fibroid and with less cost and low complication rate.

Two-dimensional ultrasound with installation of sterile physiological saline in the endometrial cavity called sonohysterography is an established technique that allows the visualization of intracavitary lesions such as submucosal myomas with a higher precision than conventional two-dimensional ultrasound and comparable to that of diagnosis hysteroscopy. In addition, SHG allows an accurate assessment of the number of fibroids, measurement of fibroid size, and the thickness of the overlying myometrium, which is called the myometrial free margin.

The myometrial free margin is a limiting factor for safe myoma resection during hysteroscopic myomectomy, but we can fix this problem by taking advantage of the contractile capacity of the myometrium with different pressure changes of the distension medium [24].

3.3 Classification: fibroid types 0, 1, and 2

In 1993, in the face of the surgical complexity posed by some deeply penetrating submucosal myomas, Wamsteker et al. proposed a classification system for submucosal fibroids to predict the difficulty of the surgical procedure, depending on the penetration degree of the fibroid in the myometrium. With this classification, gynecologists can estimate the likelihood of completing the hysteroscopic removal of the submucosal fibroid in a single procedure. The Wamsteker classification was adopted by the European Gynecological Endoscopy Society (ESGE) and the leiomyoma classification system of the International Federation of Gynecology and Obstetrics (FIGO) includes the Wamsteker classification for submucosal fibroids, depending on the penetration degree of the fibroid in the myometrium, the fibroid will form an angle with the uterine cavity: Type 0 = fibroids attached to the cavity by a narrow pedicle, Type 1 = fibroids with an angle of less than 90° with the adjacent uterine wall, Type 2 = fibroids forming an angle of 90° or more with the adjacent uterine wall (**Figure 5**).

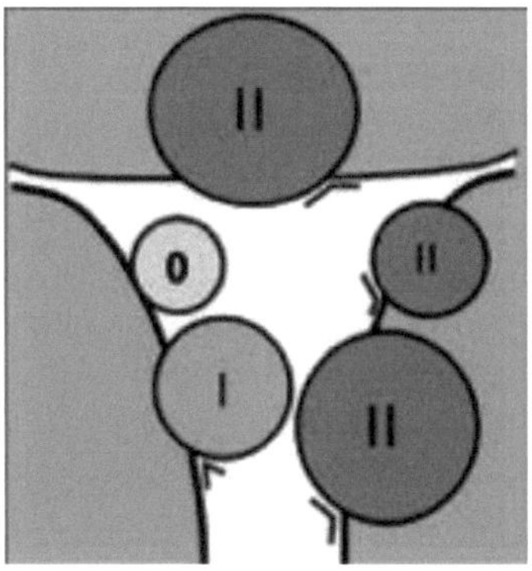

Figure 5.
Wamsteker and ESGE classification depending depth myometrial penetration.

4. Therapeutic approach

Should we treat all submucosal fibroids in the same way?

The approach to G0 fibroids with pedicles and without an intramural component should be different from G1-G2 fibroids that have an intramural component. We need to standardize the therapeutic approach to fibroids and follow pre-established guidelines [19, 25, 26].

4.1 Approach to fibroid type 0

It is recommended to cut the vascular pedicle and then the extract the fibroid with forceps, morcellation, vaporization, etc. These options depend on the size of the fibroid. Some authors recommend leaving the fibroma fragments inside the uterine cavity, which will be expelled naturally after several menstrual cycles.. There are other authors who advise against it due to bleeding and colicky pain until expulsion. A preliminary biopsy will always be necessary, if left" in situ" until its expulsion.

4.2 Approach to fibroid types 1 and 2

The general principle for a correct myomectomy is the enucleation of the fibroid; for that purpose, we must find the correct plane and that is the pseudo-capsule plane. Enucleation of the fibroid through the pseudocapsule allows for preservation of the neurovascular network of the myoma, rich in neuropeptides and neurotransmitters, which are important for a correct healing of the affected myometrium. When cutting at the correct plane of the pseudocapsule, we find lax bridges of connecting tissue and multiple capillaries or small vessels. Dissecting this plane is easy due to its laxity, and it progressively detaches from the fibroid while its irrigation becomes compromised by cutting off the surrounding irrigation. Dissection of the correct layer decreases bleeding during surgery.. Another benefit of retaining its plane is the preservation of the integrity of the underlying myo-metrium, thus preventing scars. Scars on the myometrium affect fertility after the procedure and contribute to the formation of post-surgical adhesions.

There are different techniques to approach the pseudocapsule, but in all of them we have to weaken the endometrial surface that covers the fibroid and that contains it within the intramural plane, we must weaken it to allow the fibroid to protrude into the uterine cavity, helped by the pressure changes of the median distensor and physiological myometrial contraction. The technique to address fibroids will depend on the intracavitary component:

On the one hand, if the fibroid has a small intracavitary component, we can choose one of the following techniques: all of them involve making an incision in the endometrial lining of the fibroid and promote the protrusion of the fibroid inside the uterine cavity. We can remove the fibroid in one or two step.

Bettochi technique (OPPIuM). this incision is made on the line **of the reflection of the fibroid** with uterine wall.

Myomectomy in toto. In this technique the incision is elliptical.

On the other hand, if the fibroid has a large intracavitary component, first we resect this component, then to perform the enucleation of the pseudocapsule and lastly remove the rest of fibroid, using the following techniques:

Mazzon technique. Also known as the "Cold loop" technique, developed by Mazzon in 1995, it uses monopolar or bipolar electrodes by slicing the intracavitary component and the Cold loop. It is a mechanical instrument to perform the enucle-ation of the pseudocapsule.

This technique is characterized by a sequence of three different operational steps:

First, the intracavitary portion of the fibroid is cut by repeated and progressive steps of a semicircular monopolar cut. This action stops at the plane of the endometrial surface so that the passage between the fibroid and the adjacent myometrium are clearly identified (pseudocapsule). Second, cold enucleation of the intramural portion of the fibroid is performed by pulling and lever maneuvers with non-electrical "cold" loops. Once the intracavitary portion is resected, the usual cutting loop is replaced on the same resectoscope using a suitable cold loop blunt dissection. By gentle traction on the fibroid, the pseudocapsule is clearly identified and the cold loops are then inserted into this avascular space. These loops are progressively used in a mechanical form that hooks and lacerates the connective bridges that join the fibroid to normal tissue.

Lastly, the removal of the enucleated intramural portion is completed by progressive cutting, being completely dislocated and therefore safely treatable as a lesion with a total intracavitary development which can thus be completely and safely excised by standard progressive excision using an angled cutting loop [27].

Hydromassage Technique. It changes the distention pressures of the uterine cavity, which achieves the same effect as the mechanical instruments such as Cold loop and Tissue Removal device (TRD).

Hydromorcellation Technique: Maneuvers combined with the TRD and the irrigation system (continuous infusion pump) are performed to distend the intrauterine cavity, making changes in intrauterine pressure with rises and falls of flows that will favor myometrial contractions.

The objective of this combined technique is to weaken the endometrial surface that lines the fibroid and thus allow the fibroid to protrude into the cavity. To weaken the endometrial surface that covers the fibroid, we will use the TRD and to promote the protrusion of the fibroid into the uterine cavity with the contractions of the myometrium, we will perform "hydromassage maneuvers" with changes in the flow of intrauterine distension.

We will approach the TRD to the surface that covers the fibroma, either in its upper pole or in the cleavage plane of the fibroid with the uterine cavity and once this surface has been weakened, we will perform maneuvers to change the intrauterine distension, lowering and raising the pressures of flow, even stopping the procedure for 1 or 2 minutes, in cases of fibroids with a large intramural component.

With these innovative maneuvers to change intrauterine pressure, we promote contractions of the myometrium and allow the myoma to protrude into the cavity, visualizing the plane of the pseudocapsule and its bridges and proceeding to morcellate the intracavitary portion that protrudes from the intramural portion of the myoma [28].

4.3 On-site hysteroscopy

There are many centers where hysteroscopy, even diagnostic hysteroscopy, is commonly performed with general anesthesia in the operating room. In reality, while it is a challenge to perform hysteroscopy in an outpatient setting, it is even harder to convince gynecologists around the world, who are still performing this procedure as a surgical procedure that women deserve the option of a less invasive approach. While the skillset needed for outpatient hysteroscopy can be demanding, global progress in this procedure is patchy. Recommendations for the execution of an outpatient hysteroscopy [29–31].

1. The incorporation of "outpatient hysteroscopy" into clinical practice has shown economic benefits (Grade II evidence, Grade A recommendation).

2. Gynecologists should be able to perform outpatient hysteroscopy for the diagnosis and treatment of women with abnormal uterine bleeding, infertility and intrauterine abnormalities.

3. Outpatient hysteroscopy should be performed in a room of adequate size and fully equipped, there must always be an assistant/companion in the room for patient safety and privacy (Grade II evidence, Grade B recommendation).

4. The hysteroscopist must have the skills and experience to perform a hysteroscopy (Grade VI, Grade A recommendation).

5. Written informed consent must be obtained before initiating the procedure.

Moving hysteroscopic procedures outside the operating room and bringing them into the outpatient setting facilitates the logistics around hysteroscopy: they are more cost-effective, they will improve the productivity of doctors and allow for easier surgical scheduling, they will improve patient satisfaction and make recovery times shorter. In the United States in 2017, the payment for hysteroscopic polypectomy was reduced by $30 when performed in an operating room, while the payment increased by $972 when performed as an outpatient procedure. Performing the hysteroscopy as a surgical procedure will incur additional costs for anesthesia fees and hospital fees. There is a significant benefit in increasing the number of outpatient procedures.

Patients appreciate the convenience of the "see and treat" approach to a gynecological problem and often prefer to avoid the inconvenience of going through surgery and the additional risks of undergoing anesthesia. They are associated with greater patient satisfaction and faster recovery compared to hysteroscopy in a hospital [12, 32].

The treatment sequence will depend on the workflow of each department and the surgical material available. It can be done in one step –"see and treat" – or in two or more steps, depending on the complexity of the pathology to be treated.

Therefore, it will be possible to conduct a hysteroscopy in an operating room or on an outpatient setting.

4.4 Surgical devices

Technological advances in surgical devices over the last 2 decades have brought hysteroscopy to maturity in the 21st century, allowing for many outpatient procedures.

Reliable equipment is an essential prerequisite for safe surgery.

The advent of modern small diameter (less than 5.5 mm) hysteroscopes, along with 5–7 Fr miniature mechanical ancillary instruments (scissors, forceps, bipolar electrodes, e.g. Versapoint™ [Gynecare, Ethicon Inc., Menlo Park, CA, USA). U.S]; tissue retrieval systems: TRUCLEAR ™ [Smith & Nephew Inc., Andover, MA, UH. USA], MyoSure® [Hologic, Marlborough, MA, USA] have led to a paradigm shift in surgical interventions leading to procedures that were performed under general anesthesia being conducted in an outpatient setting with local anesthesia only and if necessary [14, 33].

In 2005, Campo et al. evaluated the effects of instrument diameter, patient parity and surgeon experience of pain during office hysteroscopy and the success rate of the procedure. They found that all outcomes (pain, visualization and success rate) were largely influenced by patient parity and the diameter of the hysteroscope. Compared to less experienced surgeons, those with more experience caused less procedure pain. In contrast to the use of a hysteroscope with an outer diameter of 5 mm, outpatient hysteroscopy with a mini-hysteroscope (outer diameter of 3.5 mm) was preferable. The operating hysteroscope contains a working element which introduces electrosurgical and mechanical instruments for the myomectomy surgery [34].

Working with minimal intrauterine distension pressures, sufficient for adequate visualization, will reduce patient discomfort and serious complications such as fluid overload. Isotonic solutions (normal saline) are recommended as distension medium. It is essential that all hysteroscopic surgery offices have a control system for the balance fluids during the procedure and a protocol for the management of excessive fluid deficit [35–38].

In order to perform outpatient myomectomy, these devices must work quickly but the surgeon should also be comfortable with the device that they are using.

It exists new surgical devices with small diameters that can be used for myomas in an outpatient setting, without general or local anesthesia and using different types of energy such as the Versapoint system with bipolar energy, mechanical TRDs or laser.

4.4.1 Versapoint

Versapoint® with bipolar energy system. Currently, there are 5 bipolar electrodes available on the market, three of these electrodes can be used with small-diameter hysteroscopes and they have different terminals for specific tasks. The three different terminals are: the spring (for vaporization), the twizzle (for cutting) and the ball (for coagulation), and the other two electrodes can only be used with a classic resectoscope. They cannot be used in an outpatient setting.

4.4.2 Laser

This device achieves different effects depending on the wavelength: cutting, coagulation, vaporization. The laser most commonly used in hysteroscopy was the Neodymium laser and currently BIOLITEC with Selective Light Vaporization.

4.4.3 Mini-resectoscopy

The Gubbini Mini-resectoscope which has a small diameter for outpatient procedures uses terminals with bipolar energy and different tips (ball, loop, blade) to perform the same function as traditional resectoscopes.

4.4.4 Hysteroscopic TRDs

The Hysteroscopic TRD is a hysteroscopic mechanical system used to remove polyps and submucosal myomas. It has a terminal with a side window and a mechanical cutting blade, which rotates and oscillates at the same time. It is based on a rotary tubular cutting system with mechanical energy based on suction instead of the high-frequency electric power historically used in resectoscopy.

There are two brands in the market for performing outpatient myomectomy with different diameters and speeds.

The Truclear 5.0 system was the first mechanical TRD for intrauterine pathologies approved by the FDA (Food and Drug Administration) in 2005. It has a small diameter of 5 mm, ideal for outpatient procedures without anesthesia, with a speed of 750 rpm.

The MyoSure® system was the second mechanical TRD for intrauterine pathologies approved by the FDA in 2009. The MyoSure® suite includes four devices (MyoSure MANUAL, LITE, REACH, XL) allowing flexibility to treat a wide range of intrauterine pathologies in any setting. MyoSure works at a faster speed (8075 rpm), which reduces the duration of the procedure [39, 40]. The device can be introduced via the new generation Omni scope (diameter from 5.5 mm up to 6 mm) or the MyoSure hysteroscopes (from 6.25 mm up to 7.25 mm).

5. What factors influence for a successful myomectomy?

The main limiting factor for a successful one-step myomectomy is the duration of the procedure because the volume of fluid deficit depends on it, which is the main and most serious complication in the process of performing a hysteroscopy.

On the one hand, the complexity of myomas (fibroids with intramural penetration) increases the risk of systemic fluid absorption because the hysteroscopist needs more time for the myomectomy and this type of myoma disrupts the integrity of the myometrium. On the other hand, the skill level and experience of the hysteroscopist influence the duration of the procedure [41].

5.1 Complexity of the fibroid

We must analyze all the characteristics of the myomas before performing the myomectomy: size, number, location and type (G0, G1, G2) in order to perform a successful myomectomy. Within all existing classifications of submucous myoma, the Lasmar classification [42, 43] is the most accurate, even more so if associated with the concept of CONTINENT/CONTENT proposed by Haimovich (**Figures 6** and 7).

The five parameters of **STEPW** are as follows:

1. **Size (S):** the largest diameter found by any of the imaging methods. When the nodule measures <2 cm, it is given a score of 0; if it is 2.1–5 cm, it gets a score of 1; and if it measures >5 cm, it gets a score of 2.

2. **Topography (T)**: defined by the third of the uterine cavity where the fibroid is located. If it is in the lower third, the score is 0; if in the middle third, the score is 1; and if in the upper third, the score is 2.

3. **Extension of the base of the myoma (E)**: when the fibroid covers one third or less of the wall, it is given a score of 0; when the base of the nodule occupies between one and two thirds of the wall, the score is 1; and when it affects more than two thirds of the wall, the score is 2.

4. **Penetration of the nodule into the myometrium (P)**: when the fibroid is completely within the uterine cavity it is given a score of 0; if most of it is in the uterine cavity the score is 1; and if most of it is in the myometrium the score is 2.

5. **Wall (W)**: when the fibroid is on the lateral wall, 1 extra point is added regardless of the third that is affected.

	Size (cm)	Topography	Extension of the base	Penetration	Lateral Wall	Total
0	< 2	Low	< 1/3	0		
1	> 2 a 5	Middle	> 1/3 – 2/3	< 50%	+ 1	
2	> 5	Upper	> 2/3	> 50%		
Score	+	+	+	+	+	

Score	Group	Complexity and therapeutic options
0 to 4	I	Low complexity hysteroscopic myomectomy
5 to 6	II	High complexity hysteroscopic myomectomy. Consider GnRH use? Consider Two-step hysteroscopic myomectomy.
7 to 9	III	Consider alternatives to the hysteroscopic technique

Lasmar. New classification of submucous myomas. Fertil Steril 2011.

Figure 6.
STEPW submucous fibroid classification.

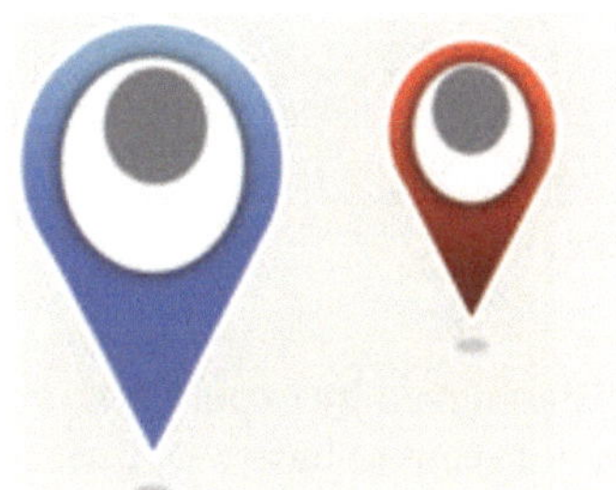

Figure 7.
The concept continent/content take into consideration the relation between the continent (uterine cavity) and content (fibroid).

Level 1
- > Diagnostic hysteroscopy with target biopsy
- > Removal of simple polyps
- > Removal of intrauterine contraceptive device

Level 2
- > Proximal fallopian tube cannulation
- > Minor Asherman's syndrome
- > Removal of pedunculated fibroid (type 0) or large polyp

Level 3
- > Division/resection of uterine septum
- > Major Asherman's syndrome
- > Endometrial resection or ablation
- > Resection of submucous fibroid (type 1 or type 2)
- > Repeat endometrial ablation or resection

Figure 8.
RCOG classification of operative hysteroscopy levels.

5.2 Skill level and experience of the hysteroscopist

While the skill set required for outpatient hysteroscopy is still state-of-the-art gynecological competence, global progress in this procedure has been irregular. Currently, entities such as the Royal College of Obstetrics and Gynecology (RCOG) and the International Society of Gynecologic Endoscopy (ISGE) have developed a ranking of hysteroscopic procedures, in terms of surgical complexity, guiding the accreditation and training in hysteroscopic surgery (**Figures 8** and **9**) [29, 31].

The resection of fibroids with intramural extension is advisable only for expert surgeons as it is technically difficult and has a higher risk of complications than other hysteroscopic procedures. Type G1-G2 myomas need a short procedure duration for

Classification of operative difficulty
Minor hysteroscopic surgery level I
Diagnostic hysteroscopy including vaginoscopy
Eye-directed biopsy
Intermediate hysteroscopic surgery level IIa
Cannulation of the tubal ostia
Sterilization
Non-embedded intrauterine contraceptive device non pregnant
Uterine metroplasty on partial septum
Endometrial ablation
Polypectomy
Myomectomy grade 0-I
Advanced hysteroscopic surgery level IIb
Myomectomy grade II
Large polyps
Resection of complete uterine septum + vaginal septum
IUCD removal in pregnancy
Extensive adhesiolisis

Figure 9.
ISGE classification of operative difficulty.

complete resection that is only achieved by expert hysteroscopists. Furthermore, the difference in equipment does not seem to have a significant impact on surgery for safe hysteroscopic myomectomy for fibroids with intramural extension [44].

6. Complications

Hysteroscopic myomectomy is relatively safe, but like any other surgical procedure, it is not without complications. Complication rates of 2% and 2.7% have been described in the literature [45, 46].

6.1 Fluid overload. Why is the operating time so important?

The estimated frequency of fluid overload is 0.2%. It is the most serious complication however not frequent; it is directly related to the duration of the procedure and to fibroids with a large surface due to the vascular damage associated to them and the subsequent intravasation of liquid due to distension. Therefore, in the excision of complex fibroids, sometimes it is better to stop and complete the operation during a second procedure. Whenever possible, we recommend the use of isotonic mediums such as normal saline. The distension mediums must be as low as possible while providing adequate distension with an intrauterine pressure of approximately 70–100 mmHg. This is usually achieved when the medium is suspended for approximately 1–1.5 min above the uterus with the current continuous pressure pumps. Garry et al. proved that intravasation of the mediums increases considerably once the intrauterine pressure exceeds the mean blood pressure (MBP). Most gynecologists have a termination threshold of 1000 mL for electrolyte-poor hypotonic mediums and 2500 mL for isotonic electrolytes.

6.1.1 How to decrease fluid overload?

There are several options to reduce systemic absorption of fluid such as intracervical injection of diluted vasopressin solution immediately prior to the procedure, the distension pressure in the uterine cavity should not be kept too high, it should be maintained below the mean blood pressure (evidence level A, stopping the procedure for a few minutes (10′) reduces systemic absorption of fluids by intravascular clotting) [35, 38]. There is consistent evidence that preoperative administration of GnRH agonists reduces the risk of systemic fluid absorption and decreases the impact of hyponatremic hypotonic encephalopathy, especially in premenopausal women [36, 37].

6.2 Uterine perforations

The frequency is low, 0.13% to 0.76%. The uterus can be pierced with a dilator, hysteroscope, or power source. Management will depend on the size, the site of the perforation and whether or not there is a risk of injury to another organ. Perforation occurs most frequently at the fundus level without significant bleeding. Simple perforation rarely causes further damage and can be managed conservatively with hospitalization, no observation, and appropriate broad-spectrum antibiotics. Complex perforation can occur with a mechanical device or energy source and therefore can be associated with thermal injury to adjacent structures, including the intestine or large vessels. However, the energy sources used in the outpatient setting are usually monopolar or bipolar energy that decrease the propagation of energy through the tissue during the process and are therefore safer. Mechanical TRDs do not require energy and continuously aspirate resected tissue through the device for better visualization and thus reducing the risk of perforation.

6.3 Intrauterine bleeding during procedure

The frequency is about 0.25%. Management will depend on the site, severity, and cause of the bleeding. Intrauterine bleeding that occurs during the procedure should be immediately obvious and can usually be controlled by spot electrocoagulation. If clotting fails to control bleeding, the procedure may need to be terminated and a tamponade applied by inserting a Foley catheter and dilating the balloon. The catheter must be left in place for 4–6 hours, after which the bleeding almost always stops.

6.4 Cervical trauma

Outpatient procedures can often be performed without the need to dilate the cervix, particularly using the vaginoscopic technique described by Bettocchi et al. However, operative hysteroscopy may require cervical dilation. Trauma can be treated with pressure, silver nitrate, or sutures. It is best to avoid over dilation of the cervix because this can cause the distention medium to leak through the cervix and around the hysteroscope.

6.5 Infection

Incidence is between 0.1% and 1.42%. Acute pelvic inflammatory disease after hysteroscopic surgery is rare. Diagnosis is made from classic signs and symptoms, and treatment should be performed with appropriate antibiotics after vaginal smear and blood culture.

7. Other frequent questions regarding the handling of fibroids

7.1 Cervical maturing

There have been studies evaluating the use of cervical "maturing" agents prior to hysteroscopy; these are typically prostaglandin analog, misoprostol, progesterone antagonist, mifepristone, or osmotic stents (laminaria stents). The literature available does not demonstrate any benefit in the use of ceramic preparations for patients undergoing diagnostic hysteroscopy. For patients who undergo surgical hysteroscopy and cervical dilation beyond 5 mm in diameter, these agents may be especially beneficial in premenopausal women [47, 48].

7.2 Paracervical block

Most outpatient procedures do not require analgesics or anesthesia, but if the patient needs any of them, paracervical anesthesia is better. According to the Cochrane database publication, anesthesia with paracervical block can decrease pain during the procedure and 30 minutes afterwards [49], while the French guidelines [50] do not recommend the use of analgesics or anesthesia to conduct outpatient hysteroscopy; in England, analgesics are administered by 62.5% of physicians [51].

7.3 Antibiotic prophylaxis

There are no studies that show any evidence to indicate antibiotic prophylaxis in hysteroscopies.

8. Adhesions

Intrauterine adhesions are frequent, especially after a myomectomy if the plane of the pseudocapsule is not respected or when two fibroids are located on opposite uterine walls; in this case, it is preferable to perform the myomectomy in multiple stages to avoid the formation of adhesions. The use of non-electrical devices (cold loop or mechanical TRDs) reduces intrauterine adhesions. Different safe and effective strategies reduce intrauterine adhesions after hysteroscopic myomectomy: early second revision hysteroscopy, barrier methods and, in particular, the barrier of non-adhesive gels, insertion of an intrauterine device and 2 months of estrogen and progestin therapy (in the form of combined oral contraceptives) [45, 52].

9. Future expectation

9.1 Should we treat small asymptomatic submucosal fibroids in patients who want to become?

Small myomas, given that they are benign hormone-dependent tumors, have a high growth potential and become symptomatic or cause complications during natural or assisted conception and pregnancy. Physicians must always take into account the biological effects of hormonal changes and/or high levels of estrogen during the reproductive life of a woman.

Even if a submucous myoma is small, it may affect the implantation potential of an embryo due to the changes produced in the myometrium, or just by causing mechanical compression.

Given that myomas are usually spherical, linear growth in the diameter of a myoma corresponds to the squared growth in surface and the cubic growth in volume [53].

The Global Congress on Hysteroscopy Scientific Committee [54] recommends the following:

When immediate fertility is not desired and in the presence of 1 asymptomatic submucous myoma smaller than 15 mm, hysteroscopic myomectomy is recommended, but expectant management is acceptable. If expectant management is favored, clinical surveillance of symptoms and serial transvaginal pelvic ultrasounds to monitor growth of the myomas are recommended.

When immediate fertility is a priority and in the presence of 1 asymptomatic submucous myomas 15 mm, hysteroscopic myomectomy is recommended.

9.2 Hysteroscopic resection of myoma type 3 (FIGO classification), is it feasible?

Type 3 fibroids are intramural fibroids in contact with the endometrium, but lack deformation of the cavity. There is no guideline for this type of fibroids. A primary goal of treating fibroid type 3 by hysteroscopic resection is to avoid open or laparoscopic myomectomy.. Hysteroscopic resection is a potential alternative to traditional surgery for this type of fibroids. This procedure should be limited to expert surgeons because it is a difficult procedure. These fibroids are not visible within the uterine cavity, but can be located by ultrasound at the beginning of surgery and resected with one of the techniques described in this chapter. The choice of hysteroscopic technique depends mainly on the intramural extension of the myoma, as well as personal experience and the available technique. The ultrasound guide is the main element to guide a safe resection [55].

10. Conclusions

Submucosal fibroids are a health problem for women and a great economic burden for National Health Systems (NHS). Nowadays, hysteroscopic myomectomy is the most cost-effective treatment because it can be performed on an outpatient setting. This type of minimally invasive surgery requires skill and an experienced hysteroscopist and new generation devices.

Acknowledgements

My acknowledgments to my great friend and artist Luisa Berlanga Solis for her magnificent drawings made for this chapter.

Conflict of interest

The author declares no conflict of interest.

Notes/thanks/other declarations

Gratefulness to my husband and **my little fairy Alba** for their love and support for the realization of this chapter.

Nomenclature

AUB	abnormal uterine bleeding
FIGO	International Federation of Gynecology and Obstetrics

RCOG	Royal College of Obstetrics and Gynecology
ISGE	International Society of Gynecologic Endoscopy
SHG	sonohysterography
TRD	tissue removal device
MBP	mean blood pressure
NHS	National Health Systems

Author details

Cinta Vidal Mazo
Department of Obstetrics and Gynecology, University Hospital of Huelva, Ronda Norte s/n, Huelva, Spain

*Address all correspondence to: zividama@gmail.com

References

[1] Machaon M. Bonafede, Scott K. Pohlman, Jeffrey D. Miller Ellen Thiel, Kathleen A. Troeger, and Charles E. Miller, Women with Newly Diagnosed Uterine Fibroids: Treatment Patterns and Cost Comparison for Select Treatment Options. HEALTH MANAGEMENT Volume 21, Supplement 1, 2018 Mary Ann Liebert, Inc.DOI: 10.1089/pop.2017.0151

[2] Anne H. Cain-Nielsen, James P. Moriarty, Elizabeth A. Stewart, and Bijan J. Borah. Cost-Effectiveness of Uterine-Preserving Procedures for the Treatment of Uterine Fibroid Symptoms in the United States J Comp Eff Res. 2014 September; 3(5): 503-514. doi:10.2217/cer.14.32.

[3] Haya Al-Fozan Joanne Dufort, Marilyn Kaplow, David Valenti, and Togas Tulandi. Cost analysis of myomectomy, hysterectomy, and uterine artery embolization. Am J Obstet Gynecol 2002;187:1401-4

[4] Marek Lisiecki, Maciej Paszkowski, Sławomir Woźniak. Fertility impairment associated with uterine fibroids – a review of literature. Menopause Rev 2017; 16(4): 137-140 .REVIEW PAPER. DOI: https://doi.org/10.5114/pm.2017.72759

[5] G Christopoulos,A Vlismas, R Salim, R Islam,G Trew,S Lavery Fibroids that do not distort the uterine cavity and IVF success rates: an observational study using extensive matching criteria. BJOG 2017;124:615-621. http:// dx.doi.org/10.1111/1471-0528.14461.

[6] Xiaoxiao Catherine Guo, B.S. and James H. Segars. The Impact and Management of Fibroids for Fertility: an evidence-based approach. Obstet Gynecol Clin North Am. 2012 December; 39(4):521-533. doi:10.1016/j.ogc.2012.09.005.

[7] Thubert T, Foulot H, Vinchant M, Santulli P, Marzouk P, Borghese B, et al. Surgical treatment: myomectomy and hysterectomy; endoscopy: a major advancement. Best Pract Res Clin Obstet Gynaecol [Internet] 2016;34(July) 104-21. Available from: https://linkinghub.elsevier.com/retrieve/pii/S152169341630027X.

[8] DonnezJ,DolmansM-M.Uterine fibroid management: from the present to the future. Hum Reprod Update [Internet] 2016;22(November (6))665-86 Available from: https://academic.oup.com/humupd/article-lookup/doi/10.1093/humupd/dmw023.

[9] Laughlin-Tommaso SK. Alternatives to hysterectomy. Obstet Gynecol Clin North Am [Internet] 2016;43(September (3))397-413. Available from: https://linkinghub.elsevier.com/retrieve/pii/S0889854516300031.

[10] Karolina Piecak, Paweł Milart. Hysteroscopic myomectomy. Menopause Rev 2017; 16(4): 126-128. DOI: https://doi.org/10.5114/pm.2017.72757

[11] Chih-Feng Yen , Hung-Hsueh Chou, Hsien-Ming Wu, Chyi-Long Lee, Ting-Chang Chang. Effectiveness and appropriateness in the application of office hysteroscopy. Review Article

[12] Christina Alicia Salazar, Keith Isaacson. Office Operative Hysteroscopy – an Update. Journal of Minimally Invasive Gynecology -2017

[13] ACOG COMMITEE OPINION. The Use of Hysteroscopy for the Diagnosis and Treatment of Intrauterine Pathology. American college of Obstetricians and Gynecologist. Replaces Technology Assessment Number 13, September 2018

[14] Natalie AM Cooper MBChB,T Justin Clark MD, MRCOG, Ambulatory hysteroscopy. The Obstetrician & Gynaecologist 2013;15:159-66. DOI: 10.1111/TOG.12039

[15] Bakour SH, Jones SE, O'Donovan P. Ambulatory hysteroscopy: evidence-based guide to diagnosis and therapy. Best Pract Res Clin Obstet Gynaecol [Internet] 2006;20(December (6))953-75. Available from: https://linkinghub.elsevier. com/retrieve/pii/S1521693406000678.

[16] Phyllis C. Leppert, William H. Catherino and James H. Segars. A new hypothesis about the origin of uterine fibroids based on gene expression profiling with microarrays. *Am J Obstet Gynecol*. 2006 August ; 195(2): 415-420. doi:10.1016/j.ajog.2005.12.059.

[17] Andrea Tinelli .Uterine Fibroid Pseudocapsule: an Update of its Importance in Fibroid Management and Female Reproduction International journal of Gynecological, Obstetrical, and Reproductive Medicine Research Vol.1 No.1 2014. http://www.researchpub.org/journal/ijgormr/ijgormr.htm

[18] Andrea Tinelli, Antonio Malvasi,Brad S. Hurst, Daniel A. Tsin,Fausto Davila, Guillermo Dominguez, Domenico Dell'edera, Carlo Cavallotti, Roberto Negro, Sarah Gustapane, Chris M. Teigland, Liselotte Mettler. Surgical Management of Neurovascular Bundle in Uterine Fibroid Pseudocapsule JSLS (2012)16:119-129 DOI: 10.4293/108680812X13291597716302

[19] Attilio Di Spiezio Sardo, Ivan Mazzon' Silvia Bramante, Stefano Bettocchi' Giuseppe Bifulco, Maurizio Guida and Carmine Nappi·Hysteroscopic myomectomy: a comprehensive review of surgical techniques. Human Reproduction Update, Vol. 14, No.2 pp. 101-119, 2008. doi:10.1093/humupd/dmm041 Advance Access publication December 6, 2007

[20] Batra et al. Hysteroscopic myomectomy. Obstet Gynecol Clin N Am 31 (2004) 669-685 doi:10.1016/j.ogc.2004.06.003

[21] Tarita Pakrashi. New hysteroscopic techniques for submucosal uterine fibroids Curr Opin Obstet Gynecol 2014, 26:308-313.DOI:10.1097/GCO.0000000000000076, August 2014

[22] Chris Sutton. Hysteroscopic surgery. Best Practice & Research Clinical Obstetrics and Gynaecology Vol. 20, No. 1, pp. 105-137, 2006 doi:10.1016/j.bpobgyn.2005.10.002.available online at http://www.sciencedirect.co

[23] Vilos GA, Abu-Rafea B. New developments in ambulatory hysteroscopic surgery. Best Pract Res Clin Obstet Gynaecol [Internet] 2005;19(August (5)) 727-42. Available from: http://www.ncbi.nlm.nih.gov/pubmed/16126460.

[24] Sherif M.M. Negm , Rasha A. Kamel, Mohamad Momtaz, Ahmed M. Magdi,Hamdy S. Azab Correlation between three dimensional multi-slice sonohysterography and hysteroscopy in the diagnosis and classification of submucous myomas. Middle East Fertility Society Journal.Volume 15, Issue 3, July 2010, Pages 209-215. https://doi.org/10.1016/j.mefs.2010.07.004

[25] Cinta Vidal Mazo, Carmen Forero Díaz, Consol Plans Carbonell. Alternative Techniques for Office Myomectomy: What Are the Limits?.In: Andrea Tinelli, Luis Alonso Pacheco, Sergio Haimovoch, editors. Hysteroscopy. https://doi.org/10.1007/978-3-319-57559-9 ISBN 978-3-319-57558-2 .ISBN 978-3-319-57559-9

[26] Karolina Piecak, Paweł Milart. Hysteroscopic myomectomy. Menopause Rev 2017; 16(4): 126-128. DOI: https://doi.org/10.5114/pm.2017.72757

[27] Francesco Paolo Giuseppe Leone, Stefania Calabrese,Carmelo Marciante, Irene Cetin, Enrico Ferrazzi. Feasibility and long-term efficacy of hysteroscopic myomectomy for myomas with intramural development by the use of non-electrical "cold" loops. Gynecol Surg (2012) 9:155-161DOI 10.1007/s10397-011-0706-4)

[28] Cinta Vidal Mazo. Obstetrics and Gynecology Service. Hospital Juan Ramon Jimenez. Huelva, Spain. Original Article "Hysteroscopic Hydromorcellation" A technique to treat fibroids with intramural component. www.hysteroscopy.info. Mar-Apr 2018 | vol. 4 | issue 2

[29] Royal College of Obstetricians and Gynecologists. Best practice in outpatient hysteroscopy. Green-top guideline no. 59. London: Royal College of Obstetricians and Gynecologists; 2011.

[30] 41st AAGL. A Practical Guide for Hysteroscopy in the Office (Didactic). AAGL 2012

[31] Practical guideline in office hysteroscopy promoted by "Italian Society of Gynecological Endoscopy" (SEGI)

[32] ACOG COMMITEE OPINION. The Use of Hysteroscopy for the Diagnosis and Treatment of Intrauterine Pathology. American college of Obstetricians and Gynecologist. Replaces Technology Assessment Number 13, September 2018

[33] Cinta Vidal Mazo. Obstetrics and Gynecology Service. Hospital Juan Ramon Jimenez. Huelva, Spain. Original Article Requirements for a successful in office hysteroscopy practice. www.hysteroscopy.info. May-Jun 2020 | Vol. 6 | Issue 3

[34] Campo R, Molinas CR, Rombauts L, et al. Prospective multicentre randomized controlled trial to evaluate factors influencing the success rate of office diagnostic hysteroscopy. Hum Reprod 2005;20:258e63.

[35] Munro MG, Storz K, Abbott JA, et al. AAGL Practice Report: Practice Guidelines for the Management of Hysteroscopic Distending Media: Replaces Hysteroscopic Fluid Monitoring Guidelines. J Am Assoc Gynecol Laparosc. 2000;7:167e168. J Minim Invasive Gynecol 2013;20:137

[36] Ludovico Muzii, et al. GnRH analogue treatment before hysteroscopic resection of submucous myomas: a prospective, randomized, multicenter study and Sterility. Vol. 94, No. 4, September 2010

[37] Campo S, Campo V, Gambadauro P. Short term and long term results of resectoscopic myomectomy with and without pretreat- ment with GnRH analogue in premenopausal women. Acta Obstet Gynecol Scand. 2005;84:756e760.

[38] McGurgan PM, McIlwaine P. Complications of hysteroscopy and how to avoid them. Best Pract Res Clin Obstet Gynaecol [Internet] 2015;29(October (7))982-93. Available from: https://linkinghub.elsevier.com/retrieve/pii/ S1521693415000565.

[39] Noventa M, Ancona E, Quaranta M, Vitagliano A, Cosmi E, Antona DD, et al. Intrauterine Morcellator Devices: The Icon of Hysteroscopic Future or Merely a Marketing Image? A Systematic Review Regarding Safety, Efficacy, Advantages, and Contraindications. 2015.

[40] Cohen S, Greenberg JA. Hysteroscopic morcellation for treating intrauterine pathology. Rev Obstet Gynecol [Internet] 2011;4(2)73-80. Available from: http://www.pubmedcentral.nih.gov/articlerender.fcgi?artid=3222940&-tool=pmcentrez&rendertype=abstract.

[41] Vahdat M, Kashanian M, Asadollah S, Yazdkhasti P, Nikravan N. The effect of misoprostol on intraoperative blood loss after myomectomy. Int J Reprod Contraception, Obstet Gynecol [Internet] 2015;4(3)776-9. Available from: http://www.ijrcog.org/index.php/ijrcog/article/view/2005.

[42] Wamsteker K, Emanuel M, de Kruif J. Transcervical hysteroscopic resection of submucous fibroids for abnormal uterine bleeding: results regarding the degree of intramural extension. Obstet Gynecol [Internet] 1993;82(November (5))736-40. Available from: http://www.ncbi.nlm.nih.gov/pubmed/8414318.

[43] Tang OS, Gemzell-Danielsson K, Ho PC. Misoprostol: pharmacokinetic profiles, effects on the uterus and side-effects. Int J Gynecol Obstet [Internet] 2007;99 (December (S2)). Available from: http://dx.doi.org/10.1016/j.ijgo.2007.09.004 S160-7

[44] Lasmar RB, Xinmei Z, Indman PD, Celeste RK, Di Spiezio Sardo A. Feasibility of a new system of classification of submucous myomas: a multicenter study. Fertil Steril [Internet] 2011;95(6)2073-7. Available from: http://dx.doi.org/10.1016/j.fertn- stert.2011.01.147

[45] Lasmar RB, Barrozo PRM, Dias R, De Oliveira MAP. Submucous myomas: a new presurgical classification to evaluate the viability of hysteroscopic surgical treatment - Preliminary report. J Minim Invasive Gynecol 2005;12(4):308-11.

[46] G. Cammareri1, A. Et al. Office Hysteroscopic Myomectomy : Effective and Efficient Procedure. International Journal of Gynecology & Obstetrics 119S3 (2012) S261–S530)

[47] Shagaf H. Bakou et al. Ambulatory hysteroscopy: evidence-based guide to diagnosis and therapy .Best Practice & Research Clinical Obstetrics and Gynaecology Vol. 20, No. 6, pp. 953e975, 2006 doi:10.1016/j.bpobgyn.2006.06.004

[48] Nathalia Andrea Cerón et al. Complications associated with hysteroscopy REPERT MED CIR. 2019; 28(1):12-18. DOI 10.31260/Repert Med Cir.v28.n1.2019.872

[49] Ahmad G, O'Flynn H, Attarbashi S, Duffy JM, Watson A. Pain relief for outpatient hysteroscopy. Cochrane Database Syst Rev. 2010;11:CD007710.

[50] Deffieux X, Gauthier T, Ménager N, Legendre G, Agostini A, Pierre F. Prevention of complications related to hysteroscopy: guidelines for clinical practice. Gynecol Obstet Biol Reprod. 2013;42:1032-49.

[51] O'Flynn H, Murphy LL, Ahmad G, Watson A. Pain relief in out- patient hysteroscopy: a survey of current UK clinical practice. Eur J Obstet Gynecol Reprod Biol. 2011;154:9-15.

[52] Ahmad Sameer Sanad, Mahmoud Elmorsi Aboulfotouh Hysteroscopic adhesiolysis: efficacy and safety. Arch Gynecol Obstet (2016) 294:411-416 DOI 10.1007/s00404-016-4107-9

[53] Stefano Bettocchi, Charalampos Siristatidis, Giovanni Pontrelli, Attilio Di Spiezio Sardo, Oronzo Ceci, Luigi Nappi and Luigi Selvaggi. The destiny of myomas: should we treat small submucous myomas in women of reproductive age? Fertility and Sterility Vol. 90, No. 4, October 2008. doi:10.1016/j.fertnstert.2007.09.015

[54] Management of Asymptomatic Submucous Myomas in Women of Reproductive Age: A Consensus Statement from the Global Congress on Hysteroscopy Scientific Committee. Journal of Minimally Invasive Gynecology. Vol 00, No 00, 00 2018. DOI: 10.1016/j.jmig.2018.06.020

[55] Capmas P, et al. Hysteroscopic resection of type 3 myoma: a new challenge? Eur J Obstet Gynecol Reprod Biol. 2016;205:165-9. http://dx.doi.org/10.1016/j.ejogrb.2016.06.026

Chapter 5

Bleeding and Hysteroscopy in Uterine Myomatosis

Sergio Rosales-Ortiz, Tammy Na Shieli Barrón Martínez, Diana Sulvaran Victoria, Jocelyn Arias Alarcon, Janeth Márquez-Acosta and José Fugarolas Marín

Abstract

Uterine leiomyomas are one of the most common diseases in women. However, there is still much about them we do not know. These tumours, also known as fibroids or myomas, affect women mainly during their reproductive years, and they are diagnosed in up to 70% to 80% of women during their lives. The most relevant part of this disease is the profound impact in the quality of life of women, in the provision of health services, and on the costs all around the world. Even though, the majority of women with fibroids are asymptomatic, approximately 30% of them will present severe symptoms, with a broad range of problems such as: abnormal uterine bleeding, infertility, and obstetric complications. There are multiple factors involved in the biology of fibroids: genetic, epigenetic, hormonal, proinflammatory, angiogenic and growth factors, growth factors that are capable of inducing and promoting de development of fibroids. The leiomyoma is surrounded by a pseudocapsule generated by compression and ischaemia of the tumour towards the myometrium and is composed by multiple elements that that promote healing and tissue repair of the myometrium after myomectomy. Therefore, its conservation in the myometrium is essential, regardless of the surgical technique used. Resection by hysteroscopy can be performed in an office or in an operating room, depending on the characteristics of the fibroid, it is required a good diagnosis and experience.

Keywords: bleeding, hysteroscopy, pseudocapsula, submucosa fobroids

1. Introduction

Uterine leiomyomas are one of the most common diseases in women. However, there is still much about them we do not know. These tumours, also known as fibroids or myomas, affect women mainly during their reproductive years, and they are diagnosed in up to 70% to 80% of women during their lives. The most relevant part of this disease is the profound impact in the quality of life of women, in the provision of health services, and on the costs all around the world.

Even though, the majority of women with fibroids are asymptomatic, approximately 30% of them will present severe symptoms, with a broad range of problems such as: abnormal uterine bleeding, infertility, and obstetric complications.

There are multiple factors involved in the biology of fibroids: genetic, epigenetic, hormonal, proinflammatory, angiogenic and growth factors, growth factors that are capable of inducing and promoting de development of fibroids.

The leiomyoma is surrounded by a pseudocapsule generated by compression and ischaemia of the tumour towards the myometrium and is composed by multiple elements that that promote healing and tissue repair of the myometrium after myomectomy. Therefore, its conservation in the myometrium is essential, regardless of the surgical technique used.

Resection by hysteroscopy can be performed in an office or in an operating room, depending on the characteristics of the fibroid, it is required a good diagnosis and experience.

2. The relevant of fibroids

Abnormal uterine bleeding (AUB) refers to uterine bleeding that, by its characteristics in duration, volume, frequency, and regularity, are outside the 5th and 95th percentiles for the female population in reproductive age and non-pregnant. In such manner that range of variation in the menstrual bleeding pattern can be very wide affecting one or more characteristics at the same time.

The abnormal uterine bleeding is divided into acute and chronic — acute when, according to a medical evaluation, the amount of bleeding justifies an immediate intervention to avoid complications secondary to blood loss. It is defined as chronic when this symptom occurs persistently in last 6 months [1].

The widespread term of heavy menstrual bleeding, refers to a sub-category of AUB, and it refers to a subjective symptom expressed by the woman as the excessive loss of blood and impacts her physical, emotional and social well-being as well as her quality of life. This term moves away from an objective measurement of volume of more than 80 ml, or a specific score and focuses on the perception of the patient, therefore, it has a better clinical focus [2].

One important aspect of AUB is that it is one of the main causes for seeking gynaecological care among 5% and 30% of women in reproductive age, and approximately one third of that population will suffer from AUB at one moment in their lives, which represents high direct and indirect costs in their medical attention [3].

The aetiology of AUB is broad since various pathophysiological mechanisms are involved, requiring the physician to have an individualised approach and a clear understanding of the systematised study and treatment options.

In 2011, the International Federation of Gynaecology and Obstetrics (Fédération Internationale de Gynécologie et d'Obstétrique, FIGO), in contribution with a large group of clinical and non-clinical researchers of 17 countries of six continents, published a system and a set of clinical recommendations about AUB to provide a detailed update with the objective of standardising different terminologies and definitions used up to that date to refer to symptoms of altered menstrual bleeding and to establish a correlation with possible underlying causes, so as to facilitate research, education and standardised and replicable medical care [4].

An AUB classification was introduced, with nine categories based on the PALM-COEIN acronym, which divides causes into structural and non-structural pathologies.

Structural pathologies can be evaluated by imaging studies and/or defined histopathologically (polyps, adenomyosis, leiomyomas and malignancy or atypical endometrial hyperplasia: PALM).

Regarding non-structural causes, these cannot be detailed by means of imaging studies, these require a detailed clinical evaluation, and an appropriate physical examination supported by laboratory tests. In most cases, a diagnosis can be established, one which corresponds to the COEIN acronym (coagulopathy, ovulatory dysfunction, primary endometrial dysfunction, iatrogenesis and not otherwise classified) [4, 5].

In 2018, FIGO recommendations were updated, including clarifications on terminologies and definitions, as well as modifications in the PALM-COEIN system which include the reassignment of some entities and orientation for subclasses of leiomyomas [5].

Leiomyomas are monoclonal tumours comprised of muscle tissue of the uterus, also referred in literature as fibroids or myomas. These represent the pelvic tumour, frequently benign, more common in women in reproductive age. At age 50, almost 70% of white women and 80% of African American women will have developed at least one fibroid [6].

There are many risk factors associated with myomatosis, and these are still being described. Among these: African American race, age, delayed pregnancy, nulliparity, early menarche, caffeine, genetic alterations, obesity, a diet rich in red meat and, recently discovered, the crucial role of progesterone and its receptors in pathophysiology, growth and development of these tumours [7, 8].

Even though myomatosis has a high prevalence in women, most of them are asymptomatic and are diagnosed as an incidental finding in a routine gynaecological examination. The main symptom of patients with leiomyomas is AUB, referred by women as profuse and prolonged bleeding, bleeding between periods, and frequent and irregular periods. These menstrual alterations are frequently used to being accompanied by the presence of pelvic tumours, dysmenorrhoea, chronic pelvic pain, infertility, compressive symptoms, and obstetric complications.

Other relevant aspects in the detriment of the quality of life of women with myomatosis are a negative impact in their sex life (42.9%), bad performance at work (27.7%), and impaired couple and family relations (27.2%). In this way, a third of women with leiomyomas will seek medical attention. Symptomatic cases will depend on size, number, and localisation of these [7, 9].

Several uterine fibroids classifications have been described. Most of them have considered the degree of extension in the myometrium and/or the distortion of the uterine cavity. Currently, this has changed, and several factors are considered in order to establish a better therapeutic approach, its possibility of success, the complete removal of fibroids and lower risk of complications.

The classification adopted by the ESGE (European Society for Gynaecological Endoscopy) based on Wamsteker's, proposes a classification of submucous fibroids according to the depth within the myometrium, classified as: G^{-0} is an intrauterine pedunculated fibroid, G-1 fibroid is majorly in the uterine cavity or has less than 50% of penetration inside of myometrium, and G-2 is mostly (> 50%) inside of the myometrium [10].

The classification proposed by Lasmar, takes into consideration, the depth of the fibroid in addition to other characteristics such as size, placement inside of the cavity, the extension of the injury in the endometrium, and the uterine wall involved, granting a rating that gives a prognosis on the difficulty or complexity of the removal, as well as the therapeutic options for its management (**Figure 1**) [11].

Another classification that also gives a rating according to size, localization, myometrium penetration and base extension is the STEPW classification. (**Figure 2**).

The FIGO classification considers any location of the fibroids and describes eight types, as well as a hybrid class (an association of two types of fibroids). It is common for different types of fibroids to be present at the same time (depending on the site), and with this classification, a more representative "map" of the distribution of the fibroids can be made. However, this classification can have difficulties when applied to very big uteri and with multiple fibroids.

SCORE	GROUP	Complexity and treatment options
0-4	I	Low complexity. Hysteroscopic myomectomy.
5-6	II	High complexity. Hysteroscopic myomectomy, consider the use of GnRH, o resectoscopy in two steps.
7-9	III	Consider other alternatives to hysteroscopic technique.

Figure 1.
Lasmar classification.

Size (cm)	SC	Topography	SC	Extension of the base	SC	Penetration	SC	Wall	SC
<2	0	Lower third	0	<1/3	0	0	0	Fibroid in the lateral wall	Plus one to SC total
>2.1-5	1	Middle third	1	1/3 to 2/3	1	<50%	1		
>5.1	2	Upper third	2	>2/3	2	>50%	2		

Figure 2.
Adapted of STEPW classification. SC: Score. Size: Larger diameter by any image study. Topography: It refers to where the fibroid is placed in the uterus. Extension of the base: How much of the uterine wall is covered by the fibroid compared to thirds. Penetration: Depth of the fibroid within the myometrium. Wall: When the fibroid is in the lateral wall, add one point to the total score.

The FIGO classification updated in 2018 is as follows:

Submucous fibroids — those located exactly below the endometrium and that protrude, disrupting the uterine cavity in different degrees are types 0, 1, 2 and 3.

Type 0: Pedunculated or with its base on the endometrial wall, but the fibroid is completely located inside of endometrial cavity.

Types 1 and 2 require that a portion of the injury is intramural (Type 1 < 50% of the average diameter and Type 2 > 50%).

Type 3 are completely intramural but are also in contact with the endometrium. Type 3 formally distinguishes itself of Type 2 by means of a hysteroscopy, using the lowest intrauterine pressure possible to allow visualisation.

Intramural fibroids (Type 4) are completely located inside of the myometrium without protruding into the endometrial nor the serosal surface.

Subserosal fibroids (Types 5, 6 and 7) represent the mirror image of the submucousal ones — type 5 with more than 50% of intramural penetration, type 6 less than 50% intramural and type 7 is attached to the serosal surface by a stalk.

In another place (Type 8): The localization must be specified, for example: cervical, intraligamentary, and so on.

Hybrid or transmural fibroids are classified by their relation to the endometrial and serosal surfaces. In these cases, one must refer first to the portion that is in contact with the endometrium [4, 5, 12].

3. The relation between the fibroid and the bleeding

The relationship between AUB and uterine myomatosis is still not fully understood, and there is a contradiction that many women with fibroids have a completely normal bleeding pattern. However, a clear relation between AUB and submucousal fibroids is observed in the context of the degree of distortion and penetration into the uterine cavity that can generate submucousal fibroids and the possible occurrence of AUB. According to literature, fibroids (FIGO 0, 1, 2 y 3) are the most symptomatic [7].

Diverse mechanisms have been proposed to explain the relationship between the AUB caused by myomatosis, however, these do not explain clearly how all these facts are intimately involved.

Previously, the most described mechanisms were the increase in the endometrial surface and the presence of fragile and congested vascularity around the perimyome, currently, it is believed that the effect of fibroids on the endometrial function represents a change in the surface inside of the uterine cavity that is not limited to areas that cover the fibroid or fibroids. Some of these changes can have an impact in the responsiveness and endometrial implantation, as well as in AUB.

An increase in uterine vascularity with larger calibre vessels that can overcome the action of platelets has also been proposed. As well as changes in the patterns of myometrial contractility, ulceration of the surface of the fibroid, degeneration of the fibroid and venous ectasia by due to of compression of the fibroid [3, 13].

In recent years, more knowledge has been gained about complex the cellular and molecular changes associated with fibroids and the AUB, with an impact in angiogenesis, alteration of vasoactive substrates and growth factors, as well as alterations in coagulation, that highlight complex interactions among coagulation, neoangiogenesis and vasoconstriction [14].

Fibroids will behave as one independent functional unit with the capacity to secrete different bioactive factors, which generate changes in situ and produce an effect on the uterus. One of these changes is the increase in the secretion of TGF-β3 (transforming growth factor beta 3), which is involved in the alteration of the homeostatic and fibrinolytic normal pathways in the endometrium since it reduces the plasminogen activator-1 (PAI-1), thrombomodulin and antithrombin III, which could explain one of mechanisms associated with AUB — an increased quantity of TGF-β has also been related to the remodelling and proliferation of extracellular matrix that could modulate the growth of fibroids [1, 15].

Regarding the causes related to the increased in bleeding in women with fibroids, different angiogenic factors have been described, such as the vascular endothelial growth factor (VEGF), basic fibroblast growth factor (bFGF), heparin-binding epidermal growth factor (HB-EGF), platelet-derived growth factor (PDGF), parathyroid hormone-related protein (PTHrP) and prolactin [2, 14].

On the other hand, there is an alteration of endothelin-1 (ET-1) and prostaglandin F2 alpha (PGF2α), both strong vasoconstrictors that intervene in the amount of menstrual bleeding by regulating the contractility of the myometrium and the vasoconstriction of the spiral artery (ET-1) [16].

4. Endometrial changes

Understanding changes generated by fibroids at the endometrial level is very complex, since it is not only a physical effect on the anatomy of the uterus exerted by intramural and submucosal fibroids, but a significant effect in the endometrial physiology and the expression and function of endometrial genes [17].

An important phenomenon to understand endometrial changes, is inflammation. It is well established that an inflammatory component is involved in most physiological processes, specifically in the reproductive process, inflammation has direct interference with follicular development, ovulation, implantation, pregnancy, labor, and menstruation are not exempt.

Inflammation is understood as the presence of leukocytes (immune cells) of different within the reproductive tract tissue, without being associated with an infectious process. This invasion of leukocytes alters function by having specific role in local regulation.

Specific sequential changes in different kinds of leukocytes can be proven inside of the human endometrium during the different phases of normal and abnormal menstrual cycles. Leukocytes are very scarce in number throughout the proliferative phase, but significantly increase all through the secretory phase, taking into consideration that around 40% of all stromal cells in the premenstrual phase are leukocytes, mostly natural killer cells (NK) and granulocytes.

The decrease in progesterone increases the expression of inflammatory mediators, including Il-8, MCP-1 and nitric oxide which promote the recruiting of endometrial leukocytes. Macrophages and neutrophils are important in the defence of the epithelium when the epithelial barrier is broken because of any reason, for example, menstrual bleeding.

Leukocytes also have the potential to release regulatory molecules that stimulate the mechanisms of endometrial repair, consequently, so the alteration of immune cells and cytokine mediators are related to the symptoms of abnormal uterine bleeding and pelvic pain, always starting from the inflammatory process produced by the menstrual cycle, fibroids, and endometriosis among other pathologies [18, 19].

Besides endometritis and endometrial micro-erosions, vascular alterations are another important factor in the causes of bleeding and endometrial alterations [20].

From the complex onset of fibroid tumorigenesis, induced among others by the t (12-14) translocation, the deletion of 7q, $HMGA_2$ gene of the locus 12q14-q15, that, under the oestrogen-progesterone promoter stimulus, the micro-environment, growth factors with mitotic activity such as growth factor 3, fibroblast growth factor, epidermal growth factor, and insulin-like growth factor, besides promoting tumour growth, are leukocyte chemoattractans, generating an accumulation of inflammatory cells inside of the fibroid tissue and the corresponding endometrium that could affect the function from menstruation to fertility [21, 22].

Another aspect related to leukocytes is the relation between the vascular endothelial growth factor (VEGF) of intravascular neutrophils and the proliferation of endometrial cells from the subendometrial capillary plexus that develops small vessels in the capillary plexus — this angiogenic process is present alongside functional activity in the proliferative phase and in pathological states [22].

Among the effects that fibroids exert on the endometrium, are the altered genetic expression and changes in the immune environment and vasoconstrictive factors, generating from a decrease in production of transcription factors necessary for implantation, within the window of implantation (WOI) to the altered production of coagulation factors during menstruation [17].

To understand these changes, it is necessary to understand how human endometrial stromal cells (HESC) regulate the expression of the tissue factor (TF), which is the main promoter of coagulation at this level, complemented by the effect of progesterone which increases a second haemostatic factor in the HESC, the plasminogen activator inhibitor-1 (PAI-1) — if this order is altered, the stability of the stromal endometrial matrix and the vascular extracellular matrix are lost by the action of the matrix metalloproteinase (MMP) -1, 3 and 9. This increases the inflammatory activity and an uncontrolled angiogenesis, with an endometrium that loses its homeostatic and proteolytic ability, and being highly vascularised.

An increase in TF expression accompanied by decreased endometrial blood flow produces hypoxia and reactive oxygen species (ROS) induce an aberrant angiogenesis and inflammation. Hypoxia produces the release of endometrial cells' apoptosis inducers secreted by human endometrial stromal cells (HESC) [23].

An altered angiogenesis due to the presence of fibroids produces fragile, hyper dilated, thinned vessels that bleed easily. The alteration of endometrial blood flow produces local hypoxia and the generation of ROS that increase the production of angiogenic factors such as the vascular endothelial growth factor (VEGF) in human endometrial stromal cells and Angiopoietin-2 (Ang-2) in endometrial cells with a decrease in HESC of angiostatic (Ang-1) [24].

5. The pseudo-capsule

In order to understand more about fibroids, it is essential to understand the myometium as a structure comprised of bundles of smooth muscle fibres surrounded by connective tissue with a network of blood and lymphatic vessels — this is the place where fibroids grow, comprised of intertwined fascicles of disordered smooth muscle cells, abundant fibrous tissue with type I and III collagen (**Figure 3**).

During its growth, fibroids compress the myometrium forming a pseudo-capsule composed of collagen fibres, neurofibres and blood vessels. Occasionally, bridges of collagen fibres and vessels that join the myometrium with the fibroid can be formed (**Figures 4** and **5**) [25].

The pseudocapsule vessels that come from the surrounding myometrium are grouped in a vascular network and the veins surrounding the fibroid in the shape of a plexus forming the image of a "ring of fire", easily detectable with a Doppler ultrasound (**Figure 6**) [26].

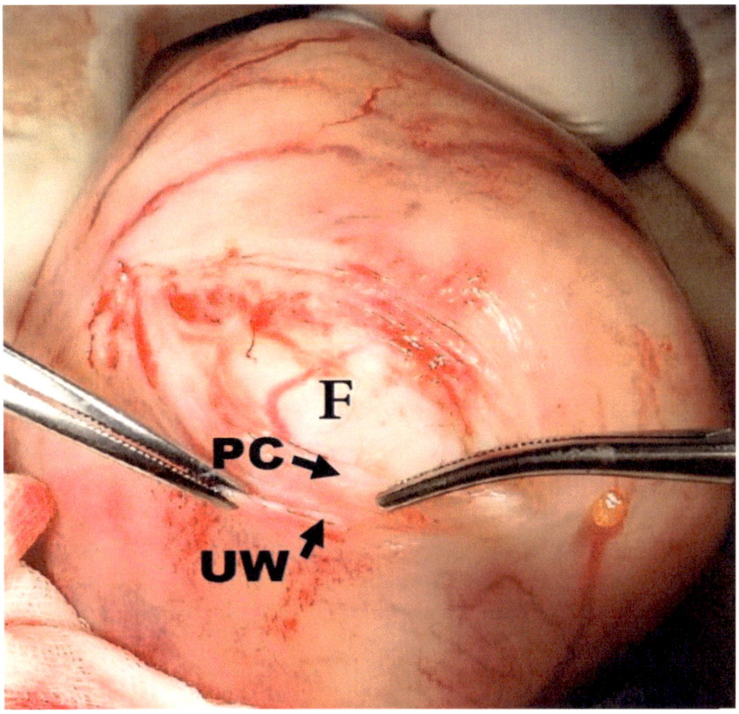

Figure 3.
Showing the uterine wall (UW) with th dissected pseudocapsule (PS) and the myoma at the bottom.

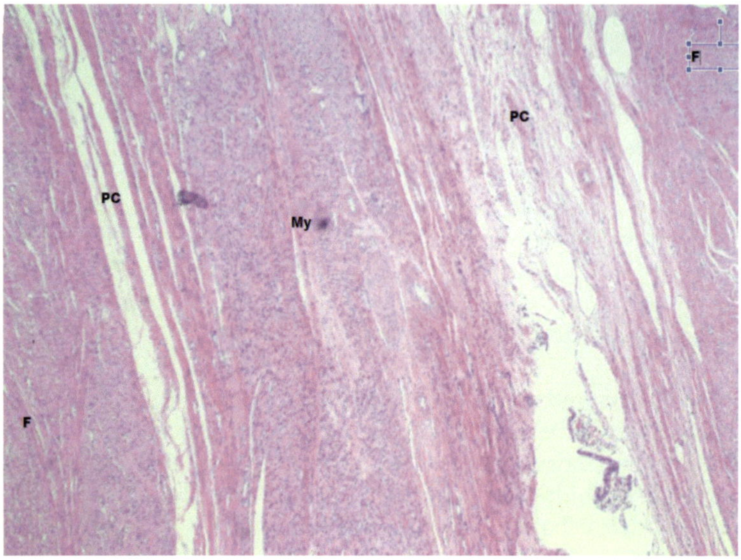

Figure 4.
Image with two fibroids at the ends (F), two pseudocapsules (PC) and the myometrium in the center (my).

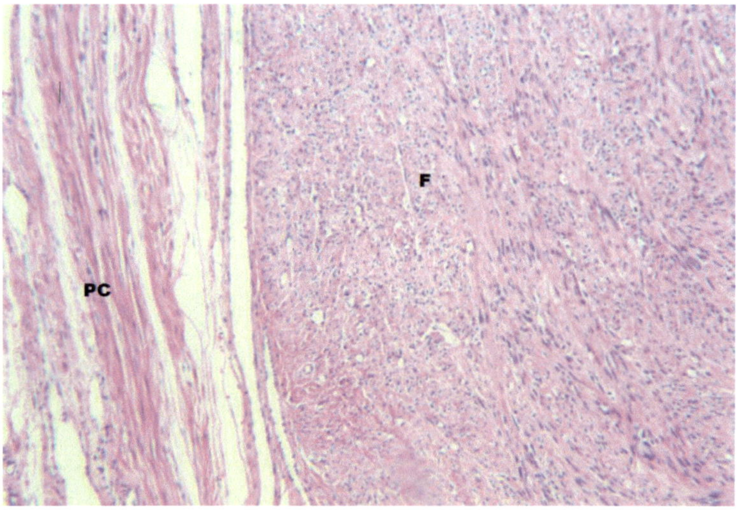

Figure 5.
Magnified image of the pseudocapsule (PC) and fibroid (F).

Angiogenesis of the fibroid's pseudo-capsule leads to the formation of a protective vascular capsule, in addition, to being responsible for the blood supply to the central nucleus of the tumour.

The biological genesis of the pseudo-capsule is not well described, however, there is evidence that is originated from the myometrium that surrounds the fibroid, therefore, the fibroid is not originated from the pseudo-capsule, but it is part of the myometrium that compresses it [27].

The pseudo-capsule is a structure rich in neuropeptides and neurotransmitters, which have a very important role in wound healing and innervation repairing besides being key in sexual and reproductive functions and being the study objective for new future treatments.

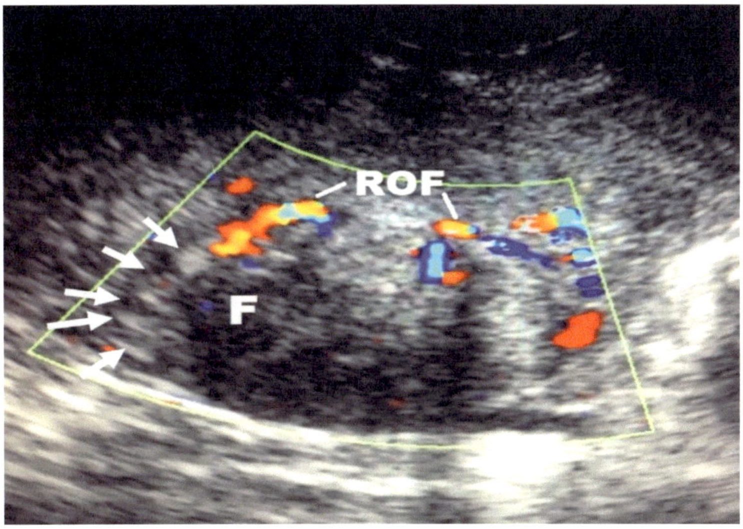

Figure 6.
Ultrasound with a fibroid in the center, with peripheral Doppler showing the ring of fire, the arrows delimit the pseudocapsule.

Neurotransmitters such as: Substance P (SP), Vasoactive Intestinal Peptide (VIP), Neuropeptide Y, Oxytocin, Vasopressin, PGP 9.5, calcitonin gene-related peptide and Growth hormone releasing hormone play an important role in the wounds' inflammatory and healing cascades [28].

The neurofibres of the pseudo-capsule contain SP and VIP just as the myometrium without pregnancy.

It is possible that these neuropeptides have influence in the physiology of the uterine contraction, cervix dilation and during labour [29].

Other research focused on the opioid neuropeptides enkephalin (ENK) and oxytocin (OXT). The study revealed the lack of positive ENK neurofibres at the bottom of the uterus and in the fibroid's pseudo-capsule in the body of the uterus, and presence of these in the isthmic-cervical area. Fibres positive for OXT were observed in the pseudo-capsule in all uterine regions, lesser at the bottom, and a higher quantity in the cervical isthmus. This indicates a larger research of neuropeptides about the impact in neurofibres in obstetric complications such as spontaneous miscarriage and cervical dystocia during labour [30].

Literature mentions the importance of knowing the fibroid's pseudo-capsule during a myomectomy, since performing a correct technique enhances the prognosis of quality of life and fertility rate in women affected by uterine myomatosis [31].

The objective of the myomectomy is to enucleate the fibroid, always preserving the pseudo-capsule. Myomectomy's technique takes prostate cancer surgery as a base, a procedure that preserves the neurovascular bundles that surround the prostate with the objective of reducing the probability of post-operative impotence and incontinence.

Taking into account these findings according to the prostatic capsule and the importance of nerve-spearing surgery, these were implemented in the surgery known as intracapsular myomectomy, preserving the fibroid's pseudo-capsule and neurovascular bundle with the objective of improving reproductive function. It is performed by coagulating, cutting, and breaking the pseudo-capsule's fibrous bridges, then extracting the fibroid directly dissecting the fibromuscular skeleton that surrounds it, always using low energy instruments (less than 30 watts). The closing of the

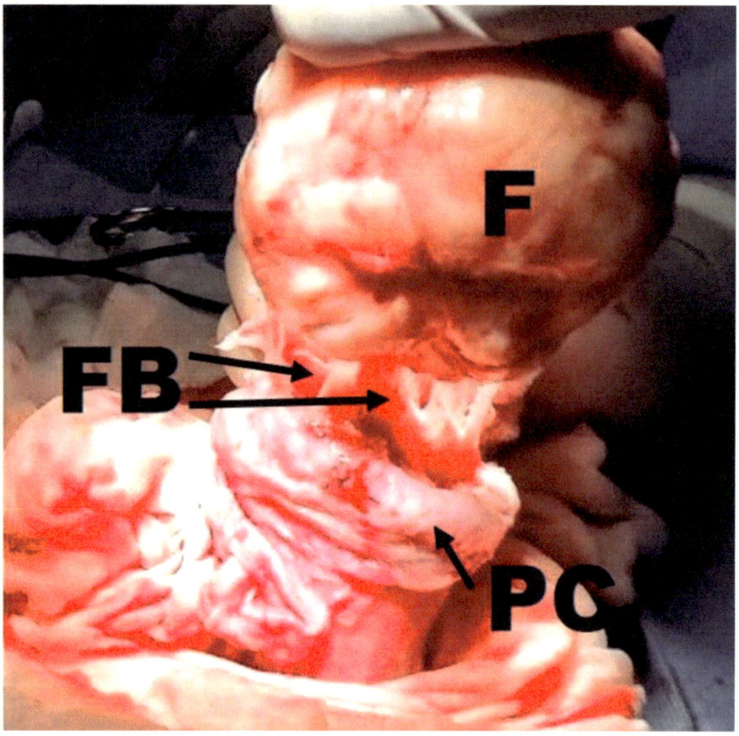

Figure 7.
Miomectomy image with dissection of fibroma (F), pseudocapsule (PC) and between fibroconnective bridges (FB).

myometrium is performed depending on the type of fibroid found — in subserosal fibroids it is performed in one plane, and in intramuscular fibroids two planes are closed (**Figure 7**). This surgical principle can be applied to all myomectomies: laparotomy, laparoscopy, and caesarean myomectomy. In comparison with intracapsular myomectomy through laparotomy or laparoscopy, laparoscopic myomectomy proved to have more benefits: lesser intraoperative and postoperative bleeding, reduced bladder pain after the removal of the Foley catheter, less use of analgesic medication and a shorter hospital stay — reduced appearance of fever, myometrial scar, bruising, ileus, and use of antibiotics were also observed during the post-operative period in comparison with laparotomy [32].

6. Leiomyomatosis and infertility

Most of leiomyomas are asymptomatic, symptoms are usually correlated with the number, size, location, and degenerative changes that these suffer — these are considered hormone-dependent. It is estimated that 30% of cases cause abnormal uterine bleeding, chronic pelvic pain and other symptoms that can affect the patients' quality of life. Leiomyomas also cause anaemia, recurrent pregnancy loss, preterm birth, urinary incontinence, subfertility, and infertility [33, 34].

The relation between leiomyomas and infertility has been a concern for a long time. *The American Society for Reproductive Medicine (ASRM)* mentions that these uterine tumours are associated with infertility from 5% to 10% of cases and are catalogued as directly responsible for infertility from 2% to 3% of patients. However, the exact mechanism, by which these cause infertility, is still in debate. Consequently, several mechanisms have been proposed to explain the possible adverse effects of fibroids on fertility, such as: alteration of the endometrial contour that interferes with implantation, alteration of endometrial blood flow that affects endometrial responsiveness, ulceration, thinning, endometrial inflammation and atrophy, endometrial biochemical alterations, triggering of uterine contractility dysfunction that alters the embryonic movement and tube obstruction. According to *the American Fertility Society Guideline for Practice*, fibroids can be associated with 5% to 10% of infertility cases, although as a sole factor, these only influence from 2% to 3% [35].

Normally, the uterus presents uterine contractions, these begins in the uterine fundus and continue towards the cervix, and their frequency increases in the early follicular phase. In the periovulatory and luteal phase, the direction of contractions is inverted, that is to say, from the cervix to the fundus, favouring the fertilisation process [36].

Fibroids as a mechanical factor is one of the simplest mechanisms that would explain infertility in this group of patients with larger and intracavitary fibroids being those that interfere in the process of transporting eggs and sperm, as well as implantation [37]. Another mechanism is through the production of cytokines and chronic inflammation — these underlying mechanisms are the ones that increase the uterine contractility mainly due by overproduction of cytokines. One study showed a considerable increase in uterine peristalsis in the presence of fibroids and after myomectomy in this group of patients, a pregnancy rate of 40% was obtained [38, 39].

The implantation process is one of the most complex and perfectly orchestrated processes in the human being. The foetal success depends on immunological changes in the mother, and it is based on modifications in the innate and adaptive immune system, in which embryo implantation and placenta development are presented thanks to immune reactions mediated by the following cytokines: TNF (tumour necrosis factor) -α and β, interleukin 1, 2, 10 and 6, among others [40].

In patients with submucous fibroids, it has been proven that a significant decrease in IL-10 and glycodelin levels, the latter being a key protein to promote angiogenesis and supress NK (natural killer) cells in the implantation process [41]. The presence of fibroids has shown alterations in the subendometrial area, a region highly rich in macrophages and NK cells. In patients with leiomyomatosis, a decrease in concentrations of these two cell populations has been proven, altering the steroid receptors at the endometrial level that are essential for the implantation process [42].

Pregnancy, live births, and implantation rates are significantly lower in patients with leiomyomatosis [43]. The presence of submucosal leiomyomas decreases the birth rate by 70%, while intramural fibroids show a decrease in the birth rate by 30% [44].

It is known that the presence of fibroids shows a deleterious effect upon the uterine contractility, depending on its location and size, particularly those that distort the submucosal and intramural uterine cavity in 60% of women younger than 40 years of age, and in 80% of women younger than 50 years of age.

One of fibroids subtypes tha most affects fertility is leiomyoma with bizarre nuclei (LBNs) which, in turn, is linked with higher concentrations of MIB1 (mind-bomb E3 ubiquitin protein ligase 1, which is an apoptosis regulator, also known as Ki-67) in the endometrium. This means, that not only the size and location of the fibroid plays a role in the subfertility observed in patients withe leiomyomatosis, but also the morphological subtype of fibroids. Furthermore, this shows that regardless of the location of the fibroids, the fertility rate was lower compared with the controls. Showing a relative risk of clinical pregnancy of 0.85 with CI 95%: 0.73–0.98 and a live birth rate with a RR: 0.69 with CI 95% 0.59–0.82 and an increase in the abortion rate with a RR 1.68 CI 95%: 1.37–2.05, in patients with uterine leiomyomatosis [45].

7. Hysteroscopical management of submucous fibroids

The coming of hysteroscopy in gynaecologic surgery has offered a new conservative approach to the treatment of pathologies of the uterine cavity.

Going back to the FIGO classification adopted by ESGE (European Society of Gynaecological Endoscopy) of submucous fibroids, describing the extent of miometrial involvement of submucosal fibroids visualised by hysteroscopy. According to the degree of myometrial penetration: submucosal fibroids grade 0, grade 1 and sometimes grade 2 submucous fibroids are candidates for this management (**Figure 8**).

The criteria for scheduling the surgical procedure must be clear, and these include a pre-operative evaluation that considers in detail the size, location, myometrial depth, distance from the fibroid to the serosa layer of the uterus, and the number of fibroids with possible degree of tissue degeneration with ultrasound or MRI, knowledge of the management of electrolytic or non-electrolytic distension fluids, and hysteroscopic irrigation pump, experience in the use of monopolar or bipolar resectoscopes, diode laser or mechanic resectors and when to select each one of them, and surgical judgement to use different techniques and to know when to stop the procedure or program it in two sessions [46].

Contraindications for a resectoscopy are: pelvic inflammatory disease or herpes infection, a distance of less than 5 mm from the fibroid to the uterine serosa, large size uterine cavity that does not allow the suitable distension and view of tumours, and a lack of surgical ability of the surgeon.

The success rate of 90% in myomectomies depends on the appropriate selection of the patient and being within the range of possible complications — from 1% to 5% in fibroids of less than 3 cm in diameter.

The entire fibroid must be removed without leaving any residual tissue and respecting the dissection plane of the pseudocapsule, which is part of the myometrium and favours the appropriate healing of the uterine wall.

The myomectomy can be performed in the office or in the operating theatre according to patient's characteristics, intra-wall extension of the tumour,

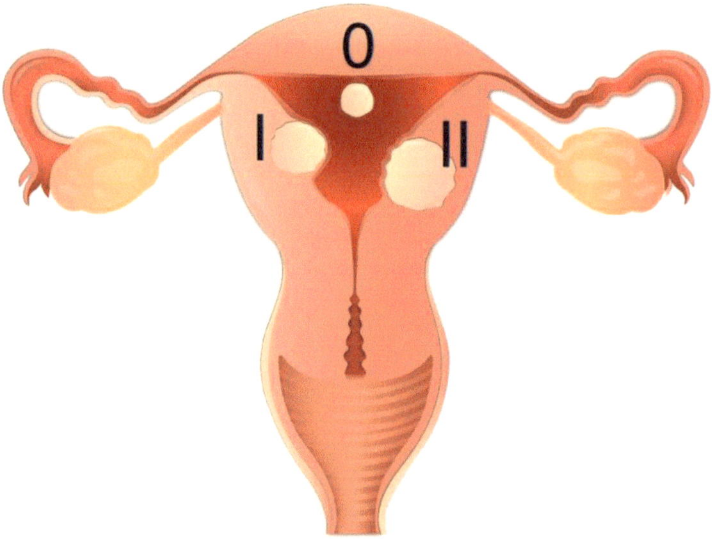

Figure 8.
ESGE classification of submucous leiomyomas.

estimated surgical time since office procedures should not exceed more than 20 minutes, the diameter of the instrument, and if anaesthesia is required to improve the conditions and results of the surgery [47].

As decision criteria G-0 and G-1 fibroids with a minimum myometrial component and smaller than 15 mm can be treated in the office. Hysteroscopic resections can still be attempted in G-1 fibroids of less than from 4 to 5 cm and G-2 fibroids of less than from 5 to 6 cm of diameter in the operating theatre and with anaesthesia since pain occurs when surgically working in the myometrium that has sensory innervation.

In order to calculate the volume of the fibroid, the V = 4/3πr [3] formula must be used.

Using a 4 mm resectoscope loop, 0.5 cm [3] is removed per minute and a 5 cm diameter fibroid has 65.4 cm [3], so on average the procedure will require two hours, being within the pertinent time limit for a hysteroscopy [48].

In the office, scissors and 5 Fr grasper clamps can be used in fibroids of less than 15 mm, sectioning the pedicle in order to extract it and, if it is not possible to, wait from 30 to 45 days for the uterus to spontaneously expel it, or the tumour can also be divided into two parts in order to extract fragments.

There is the, OPPIuM technique in G2 myomas, consisting in performing a cut with monopolar energy alongside the intracavitary fibroid's peripheral line of reflection, and in a second surgery in 30 days, resecting the leiomyoma that has emerged into the uterine cavity with a resectoscope, facilitating the procedure.

There is also the possibility of using a 45-watt diode laser with wavelengths of 980 nm and 1470 nm to cut or vaporise the fibroid with a lower rate of complications and a better vision without generating bubbles. The cutting depth is 1 mm and with special fibres, vaporisation and selective clotting of the tissue are achieved.

The gold standard is the resection with 15 Fr bipolar loop mini-resectoscope and 3 mm loop in the office and in the operating theatre, 27 Fr bipolar resectoscope with a 4 mm loop in order to completely the fibroid, while preserving the pseudocapsule. The "cut" must be programmed from 60 Watt to 70 Watt to avoid post-operative adherences. It is convenient to have the Collins loop and the cold Mazzon loops to enucleate the residual tissue, complete the surgery, and completely remove the leiomyoma.

There are mechanic tissue resection devices of different thicknesses — 15 Fr to 24 Fr with a reciprocating cutting blade and a 0 degree vision with better liquid control, that cut and aspirate the tissue by using saline solution, avoiding thermal damage to endometrium/myometrium and fluid overload. The surgeon must have the experience to align the instrument which is straight and does not allow much mobilitiy, with the fibroid in a peripheric way, and in case any vein or artery presents haemorrhage, remove the device a few millimetres from the surgical site and wait that the continuous flow clears the vision and then directs it towards the vessel and completely resects it towards its origin.

No prophylactic or post-operative antibiotic is needed, it is only used if there is a history of pelvic inflammatory disease.

The success of the hysteroscopic myomectomy depends on a personalised study of each patient and its therapeutic goals, performing a complete diagnosis both clinical and with laboratory and imaging studies including an ultrasound or magnetic resonance to perfectly locate the type and number of fibroids, their depth within the myometrium, and the distance to the serosa layer of the uterus.

Correctly selecting if the procedure can be performed in an office or in an operating theatre, because one of the main goals is the complete removal of all the tumour tissue in one or two surgical sessions, remembering that the office surgery limit is 25 minutes and that the ability to work comfortably depends on the patient's pain threshold, in addition the use of the appropriate 5 mm surgical material.

Both in the case of surgery in an office and in an operating theatre, being familiar with more than one instrument allows a better selection of the type of energy to use and guarantee the safety of the patient and avoid possible complications [49].

Author details

Sergio Rosales-Ortiz*, Tammy Na Shieli Barrón Martínez, Diana Sulvaran Victoria, Jocelyn Arias Alarcon, Janeth Márquez-Acosta and José Fugarolas Marín
UMAE, Hospital de Gineco Obstetricia No. 4 "Luis Castelazo Ayala", Mexican Institute of Social Security, Mexico City, Mexico

*Address all correspondence to: dr.sergiorosalesortiz@gmail.com

References

[1] Fraser IS, Critchley HO, Broder M, Munro MG. The FIGO recommendations on terminologies and definitions for normal and abnormal uterine bleeding. Semin Reprod Med 2011;29(5):383-390.

[2] Chodankar R, Critchley HOD. Biomarkers in abnormal uterine bleeding, Biol Reprod 2019;101(6): 1155-1166.

[3] Whitaker L, Critchley HO. Abnormal uterine bleeding. Best Pract Res Clin Obstet Gynaecol 2016;34:54-65.

[4] Munro MG, Critchley HO, Broder MS, Fraser IS. FIGO Working Group on Menstrual Disorders FIGO classification system (PALM-COEIN) for causes of abnormal uterine bleeding in nongravid women of reproductive age. Int J Gynaecol Obstet 2011;113(1):3-13.

[5] Munro, MG, Critchley HO, Fraser IS. FIGO Menstrual Disorders Committee. The two FIGO systems for normal and abnormal uterine bleeding symptoms and classification of causes of abnormal uterine bleeding in the reproductive years: 2018 revisions. Int J Gynaecol Obstet 2018;143(3):393-408.

[6] Baird DD, Dunson DB, Hill MC, Cousins D, Schectman JM. High cumulative incidence of uterine leiomyoma in black and white women: ultrasound evidence. Am J Obstet Gynecol 2003; 188(1):100-107.

[7] Donnez J, Dolmans MM. Uterine fibroid management: from the present to the future. Human reproduction update 2016;22(6): 665-686.

[8] Kim JJ, Sefton EC. The role of progesterone signaling in the pathogenesis of uterine leiomyoma. Mol Cell Endocrinol 2012;358(2):223-231.

[9] Zimmermann A, Bernuit D, Gerlinger C, Schaefers M, Geppert K. Prevalence, symptoms and management of uterine fibroids: an international internet-based survey of 21,746 women. BMC Womens Health 2012;12:6.

[10] Wamsteker K, Emanuel MH, De Kruif JH. Transcervical hysteroscopic resection of submucous fibroids for abnormal uterine bleeding: Results regarding the degree of intramural extension. Obstet Gynecol 1993;82(5):736-740.

[11] Lasmar RB, Barrozo PR, Dias R, Oliveira MA. Submucous myomas: A new presurgical classification to evaluate the viability of hysteroscopic surgical treatment - preliminary report. J Minim Invasive Gynecol 2005;12(4):308-311.

[12] Laughlin-Tommaso SK, Hesley GK, Hopkins MR, Brandt KR, Zhu Y, Stewart EA. Clinical limitations of the International Federation of Gynecology and Obstetrics (FIGO) classification of uterine fibroids. Int J Gynaecol Obstet 2017;139(2): 143-148.

[13] Munro MG. Classification of menstrual bleeding disorders. Rev Endocr Metab Disord 2012;13(4):225-234.

[14] Stewart EA, Nowak RA. Leiomyoma-related bleeding: a classic hypothesis updated for the molecular era. Hum Reprod Update 1996;2(4):295-306.

[15] Sinclair DC, Mastroyannis A, Taylor HS. Leiomyoma simultaneously impair endometrial BMP-2-mediated decidualization and anticoagulant expression through secretion of TGF-beta3. J Clin Endocrinol Metab 2011;96(2):412-421.

[16] Maybin JA, Critchley HO. Menstrual physiology: implications for endometrial

pathology and beyond. Hum Reprod Update 2015;21(6):748-761.

[17] Ikhena DE, Bulun SE. Literature Review on the Role of Uterine Fibroids in Endometrial Function. Reproductive Sci 2018;25(5):635-643.

[18] Berbic M, Ng CHM, Fraser IS. Inflammation and endometrial bleeding. Climacteric 2014;17Suppl2:47-53.

[19] Maybin JA, Critchley HO, Jabbour HN. Inflammatory pathway in endometrial disorders. Mol Cell Endocrinol 2011;335(1):42-51.

[20] Ferenczy A. Pathophysiology of endometrial bleeding. Maturitas 2003;45(1):1-14.

[21] Laganá AS, Vergara D, Favilli A, La Rosa VL, Tinelli A, Gerli S, et al. Epigenetic and genetic landscape of uterine leiomiomas: a current view over a common gynecological disease. Arch Gynecol Obstet 2017;296(5):855-867.

[22] Gargett CE, Rogers PA. Human endometrial angiogenesis. Reproduction 2001;121(2):181-186.

[23] Lockwood CJ. Mechanisms of normal and abnormal endometrial bleeding. Menopause 2011;18(4):408-411.

[24] Schatz F, Guzeloglu-Kayisli O, Arlier S, Kayisli UA, Lockwood CJ. The role of decidual cells in uterine hemostasis, menstruation, inflammation, adverse pregnancy outcomes and abnormal uterine bleeding. Hum Reprod Update 2016;22(4):497-515.

[25] Tinelli A, Sparic R, Kadija S, Babovic I, Tinelli R, Mynbaev O, et al. Myomas: anatomy and related issues. Minerva Ginecol 2016;68(3):261-273.

[26] Tinelli A, Malvasi A. Uterine fibroid pseudocapsula. In Tinelli, Malvasi A. Uterine myoma, myomectomy and minimally invasive treatment. Springer 2015:73-93.

[27] Di Tommaso S, Massari S, Malvasi A, Vergara D, Maffia M, Greco M, et al . Selective genetic analysis of myoma pseudocapsula and potencial biological impact on uterine fibroid medical therapy. Expert Opin Ther Targets 2015;19(1):7-12.

[28] Mettler L, Tinelli A, Hurst BS, Teigland C, Sammur W, Dell'edera D, et al. Neurovascular bundle in fibroid pseudocapusla and its neuroendocrinologic implications. Exper Rev Endocrinol Metab 2011;6(5):715-722.

[29] Malvasi A, Tinelli A, Cavallotti C, et al. Distribution of substance P(SP) and vasoactive intestinal peptide (VIP) in pseudocapsules of uterine fibroids. Peptides 2011;32(2):327-332.

[30] Tinelli A, Pacheco L, Haimovich S. Hysteroscopy. In Tinelli A, Mynbaev O, Sparic R et al. Physiology and importante of the myoma's pseudocapsule. Springer 2018: 337-351.

[31] Tinelli A, Mynbaev O, Sparic R. Physiology and importante of the myoma's pseudocapsule In Tinelli A, Pacheco L, Haimovich S.Editors. Hysteroscopy. Springer, 2018: 337-351.

[32] Tinelli A, Malvasi A, Hurst BS, Tsin DA, Davila F, Dominguez, et al. Surgical Management of Neurovascular Bundle in uterine fibroid pseudocapsule. JSLS 2012;16(1):119-129.

[33] Hernández VM, Valerio-Castro E, Valdez ZCL, Barrón VJ, Luna RRM. Miomatosis uterina: implicaciones en la salud reproductiva. Ginecol Obstet Mex 2017;85(9):611-633.

[34] Ramos-Ramos JA, Flores AJD, Hernández-Álvarez C, et al. Miomatosis

uterina en pacientes infértiles: descripción de un grupo poblacional y experiencia de seis años. Acta Med 2015;13(2):92-96.

[35] Lisiecki M, Paszkowski M, Woźniak S. Fertility impairment associated with uterine fibroids - a review of literature. Prz Menopauzalny 2017;16(4):137-140.

[36] Lyons E, Taylor P, Zheng X, Ballard G, Levi C, Kredentser JV. Characterization of subendometrial myometrial contractions throughout menstrual cycle in normal fertile women. Fertil Steril 1991; 55(4): 771-774.

[37] Purohit P, Vigneswaran K. Fibroids and Infertility. Curr Obstet Gynecol Rep 2016;5:81-88.

[38] Richards PA, Richards PD, Tiltman AJ. The ultrastructure of fibromyomatous myometrium and its relationship to infertility. Hum Reprod Update 1988;4:520-525.

[39] Yoshino O, Nishiss O, Osuga Y, Asada H, Okuda S, Orisaka M, et al. Myomectomy decreases abnormal uterine peristalsis and increases pregnancy rate. J Minim Invasive Gynecol 2012;19(1):63-67.

[40] Veenstra van Nieuwenhoven AL, Heineman MJ, Faas MM. The immunology of successful pregnancy. Hum Reprod Update 2003;9(4):347-57.

[41] Ben-Nagi J, Miell J, Mavrelos D, Naftalin J, Lee C, Jurkovic D. Endometrial implantation factors in women with submucous uterine fibroids. Reprod Biomed Online 2010;21(5):610-615.

[42] Kitaya K, Yasuo T. Leukocyte density and composition in human cycling endometrium with uterine fibroids. Hum Inmmunol 2010;71(2):158-163.

[43] Vam HeertumK, Barmat L. Uterine fibroids associated with infertility. Womens Health 2014;10(6):645-653.

[44] Rackow B, Taylor HS. Submucosal uterine leiomyomas have a global effect on molecular determinants of endometrial receptivity. Fertil Steril 2010;93(6):2027-2034.

[45] Pritts EA, Paker WH, Olive DL. Fibroids and infertility: an updated systematic review of the evidence. Fertil Steril 2009;91(4):1215-1223.

[46] Mazzon I, Bettocchi S, Fascilla F, DE Palma D, Palma F, Brunella et al. Resectoscopic myomectomy. *Minerva Ginecol*. 2016;68(3):334-344.

[47] Lasmar R, Lasmar B. Limiting Factors of office hysteroscopic myomectomy. In:. In Tinelli A, Alonso L Haimovich S.Editors. Hysteroscopy Springer, 2018:357-362.

[48] Lasmar RB, Barrozo PR, Dias R, Oliveira MA. Submucous myomas: a new presurgical classification to evaluate the viability of hysteroscopic surgical treatment--preliminary report. *J Minim Invasive Gynecol*. 2005;12(4):308-311.

[49] Deutsch A, Sasaki KJ, Cholkeri-Singh A. Resectoscopic Surgery for Polyps and Myomas: A Review of the Literature. *J Minim Invasive Gynecol*. 2017;24(7):1104-1110.

Section 3

Management

Chapter 6

The Contribution of Uterine Artery Embolization as a Safe Treatment Option for Uterine Fibroids

Panagiotis Tsikouras, Anastasia Bothou, Xanthoula Anthoulaki, Anna Chalkidou, Spyridon Michalopoulos, Nistikoulis George, Ioannis Tsirkas, Fotini Gaitatzi, Selma Gyroglou, Irene Babageorgaka, Natalia Sachnova, Michael Koutsogiannis, Apostolos Lazarou, Arsou Chalil Bouratzan, Theopi Nalbanti, Panagiotis Peitsidis, Konstantinos Nikolettos, George Dragoutsos, Thedosia Vogaitzaki, Stefanos Zervoudis, George Iatrakis, Werner Rath, Nikolaos Nikolettos and Vasileios Souftas

Abstract

Uterine fibroids have remarkably heterogeneous clinical characteristics with unknown exact etiology. The treatment of fibroids should be individualized based on their size, location, growth rate, the symptoms that they cause, the desire to have children and the age of the woman. Embolization is currently the most advanced non-surgical technique. The majority of women report satisfactory post-treatment results like shorter hospitalization period and recovery time in comparison to hysterectomy and improvement or complete remission of clinical symptoms. Complications include amenorrhea (in the majority of cases: recurrence after three months) and infections that are generally treated with antibiotics. The results from most clinical studies and our published experience indicate that embolization improves pelvic symptoms related to uterine fibroids. Collaborative efforts between gynecologists and interventional radiologists are necessary in order to optimize the safety and efficacy of this procedure. In the future, embolization could be generally recommended as treatment option for women who desire future fertility/pregnancy.

Keywords: uterine fibroids, treatment, uterine artery embolization

1. Introduction

Uterine fibroids are high prevalent benign tumors that originate from muscle cells of the uterus with remained incompletely understood incidence, progression disease and natural history [1]. The above mentioned tumors may appear single or multiple but usually remain asymptomatic [1, 2]. Fibroids appear in various areas of uterus, different sizes and exist not a general accepted classification system for fibroid evaluation [3, 4]. They represent a tremendous public health problem with multiple difficulties and financial cost on society [1–4].

Treatment strategies to prevent the fibroid limit growth and non-surgical treatment are needed [5–8]. Minimally invasive methods like uterine artery embolization (UAE) as treatment option of fibroids by retaining the uterus among the women during middle or late reproductive years is the summarized goal of this literature review with detailed 12 years results report of Department Obstetrics and Gynecology in cooperation with Interventional Radiology Unit of Radiology Department, Democritus University of Thrace in Greece. The aim of this retrospective study was to investigate the contribution of UAE and the occurrence of transient, or permanent amenorrhea as well as reappearance of regular menstruation, inflammation, pain in premenopausal women up to one year of postoperative follow-up UAE.

2. Incidence

The fibroids occur in a phenotype in wide of genetic diseases, clinically not as single disease entity and their progression varies and based on the various types of disease in different national groups [9, 10]. The incidence of asymptomatic but sonographically fibroids detected as remarkably high and the incidence depending on women age and race. Their prevalence is 9% in white women, three to nine times higher prevalence in African American, diagnosed in 3.3% of 25 to 32 year olds, 7.8% of the 33 to 40 year olds and increased 20-fold to 6.20 per 1000 women years by ages 45to 50 [9–14]. Familial aggregation studies confirm heritability of fibroids 2.5 times more at risk in first degree relatives, increasing to 5.7 for women with an affected first degree relative of less than 45 years old. The grow and recur rate of fibroids after abdominal myomectomy reported as 5 year risk 62% with 9% risk an additional major surgical procedure. Relapses of 27% over a period of 10 years are reported with increasing frequency rate approaching to premenopausal period [9, 14, 15].

The recurrence risk is lower in women with single fibroid with small size and in those women who noticed a subsequent successful pregnancy. Oral contraceptives administration decreased the occurrence of fibroids depending to the duration of oral contraceptives use [16–18]. Moreover, early menarche and high body mass index (approximately 18% for each 19 kg increase) are some other factors that lead to the development of fibroids [9, 14, 15, 19]. Clinically fibroids occur at least three distinct phenotypes like: single, multiple varying size and in association with adenomyosis or alone [9]. Fibroids interfere not only with implantation but also with successful labor and if there are not existing, is for a woman more likely to be pregnant. Pregnancy prevents the development of fibroids, because is associated with fibroid inflated effect [9, 14, 16–18]. The risk of fibroids decrease with parity up to fivefold [9, 14]. Although subfertility may be caused by fibroids, however the detected fibroids during pregnancy not influence the age of delivery of the first child, but change the age of last term labor. The presence of fibroids in the majority are not associated to any symptoms but is poorly explain their contribution to symptoms menstrual disorders heavy menstrual flow or longer duration of menses, pelvic pain and infertility. Based on the published literature is demonstrated a relationship between diastolic pressure and fibroids [9, 16–20]. High diastolic blood pressures led to atherogenesis, cause injury and damage of muscle cells like a similar mechanism as in vascular muscle system, release cytokine in uterus muscle, which led to promotion of fibroid growth [9, 16–20]. Approximately 10 mm Hg increasing of blood pressure led to 8–10% increased fibroid risk. Myometrial injury based either on ischemia, hypertension or atheromatic type mechanisms are associated positively also to pelvic inflammatory disease [9, 16–20]. The risk of fibroids is low, if the estrogen levels are low and this could be explain the low risk associated with smoking, alcohol and caffeine consumption.

3. Heritable disease associated to fibroids

Some fibroids reflected genetic syndromes feature fibroids development such Reed's, Bannayan Zonana, Cowden syndrome, herediatary leiomatosis and renal cell cancer (HLRCC). Reed's syndrome is well known as familial leiomyomatosis cutis and uteri (MIM150800) is an autosomal dominant trait with reduced penetrance associated with cutaneous fibroids. Bannayan Zonana (MIM153480), Cowden (MIM158350) syndromes are autosomal dominant hamartomatous polyposis disorders included lipomas, interstinal hamartomatous polyps and various nonneoplastic manifestations [21–24].

Intracellular mutation such as chromosomal translocations and deletions are reported. None of the mentioned patterns of inheritance have been clearly proved in fibroids as a solitary phenotype.

In addition, different genetic subtypes can be found in different fibroids of the same patient. Many fibroids in a uterus may be of different cytological origin. The heterogeneity from growth and development of fibroids based on enzyme glucose-6-phosphate dehydrogenase (G6PD) isoenzyme analysis and using androgen receptor (AR) gene assays reveal that fibroids are monoclonal lesions arise independently from the same uterus and may associated to various chromosomal abnormalities which results in a distinct fibroid is a monocyte in the origin of the monoclonal independent lesion [25–28].

In uterus referred high rate of estrogen receptors, which comprised spiral linear muscle fibers separated from the natural surrounding uterine muscle tissue by a pseudocapsule of connective tissue.. Many distinct factors contribute to tumor progression [25–28].

Approximately 40% of fibroids are karyotypically abnormal which compared to normal fibroids are generally more cellular and have a greater mitotic index lower DNA content. The most prevalent types of chromosomal aberrations are as following: t(12,14), (q14-q15,q23-q24), rearrangement of 6p21, del(7)(q22q32), 1p36, 10q22, 13q21–22 nad of x chromosome partial deletion 3q, trisomy 12. [29–32]. Fibroids with abnormal karyotypes are associated to anatomically positions 12% of submucosal, 29% of subserosal and 35% of intramural. Based on low frequency of karyotypic rearrangement is the explanation that submucosal fibroids are highly symptomatic and led to menorrhagia. Further research in the genetics of fibroids is needed to investigate the heritability based on their clonal mosaic nature to correlate genotypic and clinically characteristics [29–34].

4. Adenomyosis

In UAE practice for therapy of symptomatic types adenomyosis either of pure (diffuse, focal) or mix form (coexistence with fibroids) in 70% and 30% of cases respectively depending on size and number of fibroids (adenomyosis dominance, fibroid dominance) is reported a ratio 7:2:1 between the treated women [35].

Adenomyosis is characterized by the development of ectopic endometrial glands and a stroma in the myometrium, at a depth > 2.5 mm from the endometrial-myometrial separation surface and moreover by hypertrophy or hyperplasia of the smooth muscles of the myometrium [36–39]. An older description is given by Rokintasky 1860 adenoid cystosarcoma of the uterus and for the first time by Frankl 1925 the term of adenomyosis of the uterus [36–39]. Clinical diagnosis of adenomyosis is only hypothetical, histological examination poses diagnosis of the disease after hysterectomy [36–39]. It is diffuse (adenomyosis) or focal (adenomyoma), asymmetrically affects the uterine wall of premenopausal women (usually the posterior) and often coexists with myomas [36–39]. The disease is common (5% - 70% in the surgical series, using strict criteria 10% - 18%), progressing and manifested with non-specific symptoms, which are similar to the symptoms caused by myomas (bleeding - anemia, pain, dysmenorrhea, dyspareunia, pelvic load (bulk symptoms) - sensitive uterus or a combination of the above), so it is difficult to diagnose only by clinical criteria [36–39]. An incidence of 10% -30% is described, in hysterectomy preparations it was found in a percentage of 10% - 18%. 80% of women with adenomyosis have another uterine condition like pelvic endometriosis and endometrial polyps (2% - 20%) endometrial hyperplasia, adenocarcinoma [36–39]. In 35% of women with adenomyosis do not show any symptoms and the diagnosis of the disease is random [38–41]. The pathogenesis of adenomyosis remains unknown. Etiology: According to various studies the endometrial glands of the disease express more in immunochemical examinations the ratio of HCG/LH receptors found in endometrial cancers and trophoblastic disease, compared to natural [36–39]. Other theories of pathogenesis include elevated estrogen levels, endometrial injuries in surgeries such as scraping, fibromyectomy, cesarean section, and residual of Muller Duct. Adenomyosis occurs mainly in multiparas with an incidence of 5–70%. Symptoms of adenomyosis (menorrhagia (50%), dysmenorrhea (30%), uterine bleeding (20%), dyspareunia (sporadic additional symptom) [38–41]. The clinical diagnosis of adenomyosis is only hypothetical and only histological diagnosis makes the diagnosis of the disease after hysterectomy. Preoperative transvaginal ultrasonography (TVUS) and magnetic resonance (MRI) are useful diagnostic examinations Main diagnostic TVUS criteria are as following: asymmetrical uterine enlargement, subendometrial halo thickening, indistinct endometrial myometrial border, myometrium is thickened ventrally and associated to heterogeneous echotexture. MRI is another recommend imaging examination preprocedural of UAE with higher specificity compared to TVUS approximately (86–96%)and excellent to recognize fibroids,adenomyomas if the myometrial thickness is increased or the myometrium occur anatomical area changes In focal adenomyosis occurs low signal intensity within the myometrium, while in diffuse adenomyosis appear the junctional zone diffuse thickening also with low signal intensity in T2 weighted MRI The treatment options are: Drug treatment (usually ineffective), Presence of estrogen receptors in fibroids promote the increase in fibroid size. Progesteroids such as medroxyprogesterone acetate, norethindrone in GnRH-suppressed patients may increase in size. Stimulation of fibroid enlargement is a complex process involving the interaction of estrogen-progestogens in combination with local growth factors [38–41]. Antiprogesteroids such as mifepristone RU-486 reduce fibroid size. Invasive treatment of fibroids: myomectomy (open - intra-abdominal, laparoscopic, hysteroscopic), hysterectomy, myolysis - catalysis cryocatalysis, thermal catalysis by microwave or radio frequency (RF-ablation), ultrasound focus catalysis (FUS) and laser photocatalysis] and uterine artery percutaneous embolization (UAE) [38–42].

5. Clinical symptoms of fibroids

The majority of 60–70% are asymptomatic. The clinical recognized significantly underestimates the true occurrence due to the fact that the routine ultrasound screening in not obligatory indicated [43–46].

Approximately 62% of women with symptomatic fibroids visit the gynecologists due to multiple symptoms depending on their anatomical location, (subserosal, intramural, submucosal or intracavity) size number and associated degenerative morphological changes [43–46]. The referred symptoms are as following: abnormal vaginal bleeding (most common), anemia, pelvic mass, frequent urination, possible incontinence constipation tenesmus rectal pressure, pelvic pain and infertility [43–46]. Pregnancy related fibroid behavior: growth which is reported controversy concerning to increasing or remain the same the uterus size, degeneration, pain, spontaneous abortions, obstetric complication (premature labor in 15%, intrauterine restriction in 10% and malpresentation in 20%) .[43–46]. The pregnancy in coesting of fibroids depending on their anatomical location and the distance to placental site. Other rare associations are as following: Ascites development due the transudation of fluid after torsion and obstruction of vessels in floating fibroids, Polycythemia secondary detected, familial syndromes with renal cell carcinoma, intravenous leiomatosis and benign matastasizing uterine fibroids [43–46].

The most common symptom in the majority of cases in clinical practice is the abnormal vaginal bleeding. This symptom in association with myomas occurs either as menorrhagia or hypermenorrhea, while metrorrrhagia is not typical for fibroids and need more investigation to rule out malignancies. The exact mechanism of abnormal bleeding from fibroids is not yet well known. Fibroids alter the nature of uterine muscle contractions and prevent the uterus from controlling the degree and intensity of bleeding during menstruation. The submucosal fibroids due to total or partial protrusion in uterus cavity led most likely to menorrhagia while the intramural myomas have obstructive effect on uterine vessels and subsequent led to endometrial vessels ectasia with profuse menstrual bleeding [43–46].

Hypermenorrhea occur most likely in endometritis in association to submucous myomas. The palpation of myomas based on enlarged irregular uterine contour can be useful to clinically diagnosis of fibroids and the findings described as uterus size like in pregnancy [43–48]. If the uterus size is more than 12–20 week can be palpated on abdominal examination. In cases of increased size of uterus arise pelvic pressure on adjacent organs like urinary tract, rectosigmoid with frequent urination, ureteral obstruction tenesmus due to incarceration of enlarged uterus in Douglas pouch and dysmenorrhea [43–48].

The incidence of malignant mutation in sarcomas is reported to be 0.1–0.29% of diagnosed fibroids [43, 49, 50]. Leiomyosarcoma is an independent malignant tumor in the absolutely majority and arises de novo, however recently published studies reveal that in very rare cases is possible in fibroids with chromosome deletions to develop in leiomyosarcoma most common in the 5th–6th decade of life. Γλωσσική επιμέλεια.

It is characterized by extensive abnormal bleeding and a rapid increase in uterine size in postmenopausal patients [43, 49, 50]. The main microscopic features which are significant predictors of leiomyosarcoma clinical course included: coagualtive tumor cell necrosis, degenerating hyperchromatic, pleomorphic nuclei, cytologic atypia, mitotic index MI (MI denotes definite mitotic figures (mf) per 10 high power field (hpf) MI $\geq$ 5mf/10hpf, differentiation. In case of fibroids, the MI < 5mf/10hpf no atypia and necrosis and in the subgroup of leiomyosarcoma or smooth muscle of uncertain malignant potential (STUMP) [43, 49, 50]. In STUMP tumors the main diagnostic criterion associated to prognosticate biologic behavior is the MI < 5mf/10hpf but is presence of moderate to severe atypia without necrosis [43, 49, 50]. The least subgroup of tumors is accompanied by lymph nodes in the lung or other sites with histopathological occurrence similar to the original tumor approximately 15 years after hysterectomy. Immunostaining for expression of cell cycle regulatory proteins like Ki-67,cyclins E,A,cdks (cdk2,cdc2), p16, progesterone receptors, p53 Her-2/neu based on significant elevated levels in leiomyosarcomas can be useful in discriminating and identifying STUMP tumors, leiomyosarcoma and fibroids [43, 49, 50].

6. Treatment options

The uterine fibroids is the most common uterine pathology with a prevalence more than 25% of all reproductive years and approximately 1.6 million women in United States diagnosed with uterus myomatosus. Asymptomatic fibroids could be found incidentally on pelvic imaging and management therapeutical strategy depending on their causing clinical symptoms [51]. If cases which are asymptomatic need not any treatment and after menopause due to their regression expectant management is the recommended therapy option. In symptomatic fibroids based on the most common symptoms, heavy menstrual bleeding and painful menstruation is very useful. Fibroid classification system based on the fact that the above mentioned symptoms caused by fibroids which distort the uterine cavity [49].

Fibroid classification system is referred as following:

Type 0 completely intracavity fibroids.

Type1 ≥ 50% in the cavity intramural.

Type 2 < 50% in the cavity intramural.

Type 3 intramural but approach endometrium.

Type 4 intramural.

Type 5 subserosal but at least 50% intramural.

Type 6 subserosal but less than 50% intramural.

Type 7 subserosal pedunculated.

Type 8 cervical [51].

According to Donnez [52, 53] staging, submucosal fibroids are classified as following:

Grade I Fibroids with the largest diameter in the endometrial cavity.

Grade II Fibromyomas with the largest diameter in the myometrium.

Grade III Appearance of multiple fibroids>2.

7. Medical treatment

Medical therapies based on therapeutical manipulating the fibroid hormonal environment. Steroid hormones, especially estrogen and progesterone are associated to fibroids behavior, proved by clinical molecular biological pharmacological models and play an important role to their medical treatment. The combination of estrogen progestin or progestin alone is the first line medical therapy for uterine fibroids.

GnRH (gonadotropin releasing hormone)-agonists led to down regulation of GnRH receptors at level of pituitary after initially increase the release of gonadotropins flare effect of heavy vaginal bleeding, reduce the FSH (follicle stimulating hormone) LH (luteinizing hormone) and ovarian steroid hormone and produce a hypoestrogenic menopause state [52–56]. Subsequent results amenorrhea and reduction of the size of fibroids pronounced within three months after beginning of treatment [54–58]. The reduction can reach 40–50% of the tumor in 3 months but is reversible after stopping treatment. This effect is more pronounced in submucosal fibroids due to a higher number of estrogen and progesterone receptors.

GnRH antagonists often used to treat myomas before surgical procedure, block pituitary receptors and led immediately to declination of FSH, LH levels and fibroid, uterus volume reduction within 3 weeks of therapy beginning. Their directly promptly block gonadotropin effect has rapid clinical character and is associated to initial flare effect. They are currently indicated only for ovulation induction [54–58].

The presence of aromatase in fibroids and additional to ovarian estrogen activity, interleukin 1βc AMP analoque, prostaglandin E2 led to estrogen production in fibroids cells [54–58]. Fibroids express aromatase higher levels compared to surrounding intact myometrium. In these cells occur significant conversion of androstendione to estrone and subsequent to estradiol which has full biologic activity and act positively to significant stimulation of proliferation of fibroids cells [54–58].

Aromatase inhibitors inhibit ovarian and peripheral estrogen production due to cellular proliferation inhibition, androstendione inhibition and reduce estradiol levels after 24 hours of treatment. SERMs (selective estrogen receptor modulator) are nonsteroidal agents who bind estrogen receptor and based on target tissue show estrogen agonist or antagonist effect [51, 59, 60]. While the SERM Tamoxifen has agonist effect in endometrium, Raloxifen exhibit no agonist activity and decrease the fibroid size. Antiprogesterone agents act at the level of progesterone receptors (PR-A PR-B), which are abundant in the fibroid. It is reported that progesterone induce proliferation, up regulate growth factors, antiapoptotic proteins like EGF in fibroid cells [51, 59, 60]. Mifepristone is the most studied antagonist of progesterone and due to high progesterone affinity led to amenorrhea, reduction of fibroid size and improvement the clinical symptoms [51, 59, 60]. The administration of ulipristal acetate, who is a selective progesterone receptor modulator, has proved successful effects on therapy of fibroids with clinical symptoms reduction of their size and endometrium cystic glandular changes. Danazol (19a nortestosterone derivate) inhibits pituarity gonadotropin secretion, led to ovarian steroid production and suppression of endometrial growth after 6 months treatment [51, 59, 60]. The use of progestin containing intrauterine contraceptive device (LNG -IUDs) as local therapy for menorrhagia and symptomatic uterine fibroids has been studied and confirmed a significant reduction in bleeding and fibroid size. However uterus myomatosus with a distorted uterine cavity or a submucosal fibroid is a contarindication for LNG –IUD [51, 59, 60].

8. Surgical treatment

Although the traditional treatment for uterine fibroids remains the hysterectomy either abdominal or vaginal classical, total laparoscopic assisted vaginal hysterectomy, robotic assisted laparoscopic hysterectomy as the predominant surgical procedure, however is preferred only in women who have completed their family planning [61–65].

In late reproductive age and premenopausal period available therapeutic options to preserve the uterus allow possible an attempt at conception and are surgical or conservative options. Over the past decade, the hysterectomy rate has decreased while alternative therapy options for symptomatic fibroids have been increased. The surgical procedures include myomectomy, abdominal myomectomy, laparoscopic myomectomy, laparoscopic thermal ablation, percutaneous ablative methods, hysteroscopic myomectomy, myolysis, laparoscopic morcellation and finally uterine artery ligation and occlusion performed either as surgical ligation during laparoscopy [61–65]. (παρακάτω θα μπορούσε να μπεί παράγραφος για τους κινδύνους της σε περίπτωση STUMP tu).

In cases of laparoscopic morcellation is of great importance to exclude based on evaluations criteria like presence of coagulations necrosis, no significant atypia and mitotic index ≤10 STUMP tu due to unknown malignant potential behavior. Minimally invasive therapies non-surgical procedures are as following: Magnetic resonance guided focused ultrasound ablation (MRgFUS) and UAE. MRgFUS based on ultrasound energy through the abdominal layers without requirement of incisions under real time MRI monitoring to reduce fibroid size [66]. Γλωσσική επιμέλεια UAE blocks selective the uterine artery blood flow led to shrink of fibroids [67]. The goal of this review was to report our 12 years of experience from the impact of UAE on ovarian reserve (OR) (which refer to number and quality of the follicles left in the ovaries) of normal menstruating premenopausal women and to estimate the degree of pain and inflammation caused by UAE in our patients based on AMH levels and inflammatory parameters (CRP, temperature, white blood cells) respectively.

9. UAE uterine artery embolization as treatment option

UAE to treatment of fibroids as alternative to surgical procedure was reported for first time by Ravina in 1995 [67]. This is not only treatment option for fibroids but used successfully also in refractory postpartum bleeding, or after gynecologic surgery, abnormal malignancy suspicious vaginal bleeding or in cases with uterine arteriovenous malformation. Although several reports confirm satisfactory results of treatment of symptomatic fibroids without necessity of surgical procedure based on the optimal cooperation between gynecologist and interventional radiologist, however the absolutely majority is retrospective and exist no prospective randomized trials to prove the effectiveness of this procedure compared to other therapy options [67–70]. The UAEs were performed in the Department of Radiology by an experienced interventional radiologist.

9.1 Preprocedureal management

All study participants were normal menstruating premenopausal women aged between of 38–50 years old (42.6 ± 7 years on average), had attended the department of obstetrics and gynecology of our University hospital complaining of serious symptoms of uterine fibroids (menorrhea, anemia, pelvic pain, bulky symptoms, pressure effects) underwent UAE for uterus fibromyomas and/or adenomyosis (pure or mix type). The enrolled premenopausal women diagnosed with and normal ovarian reserve as defined by AMH and FSH measurements (serum FSH concentration > 10 IU/L (on day 3 of menstrual cycle), serum AMH (2–8 pg./l). In all patients were available cervical pap smear test and previously performed fractional curettage. Exclusions criteria: Women with pelvic infection, pregnant (or willing to be pregnant) women, cases suspicious of any pelvic malignancy, postmenopausal women, women with resistant clotting disorders or severe allergy to contrast media, ovulatory problems, previous ovarian surgery, PCOS (polycystic ovarian syndrome) or coagulopathy, immunocompromised, previous pelvic irradiation or women who had been offered hormonal therapy for fibroids with GnRh agonists, were excluded. All patients underwent MR Imaging on a 1.5 Tesla (Multiva, Koninklijke Philips N.V.) or an 1 Tesla equipment (GE Healthcare, Milwaukee, USA) up to 60 days before UAE,

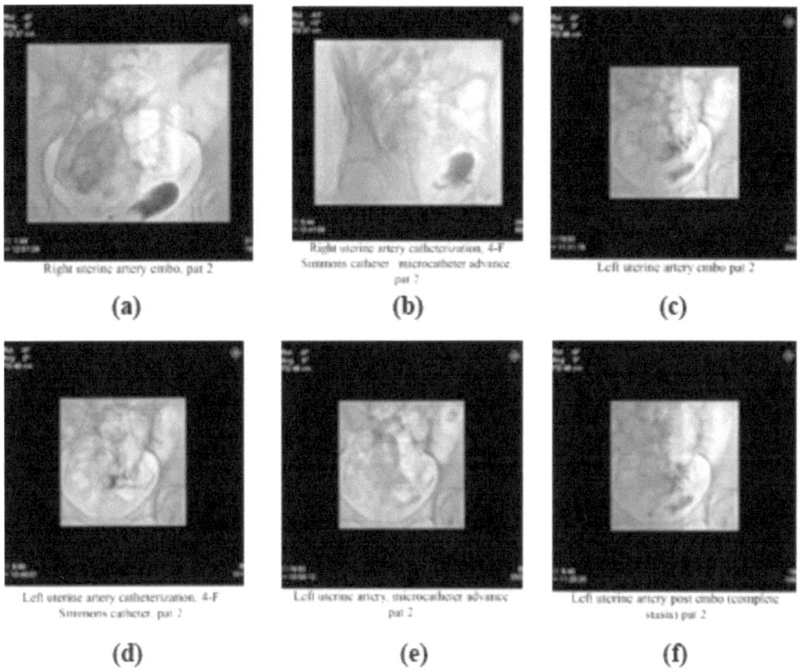

Figure 1.
Description of UAE procedure course.

using phased-array pelvic coils (**Figure 1a-f**). MR imaging included at least sagittal, coronal and transverse T2-weighted images, T2*-weighted images, T2-weighted fat saturated images, Diffusion-weighted images, T1-weighted images, and sagittal, coronal and transverse fat saturated T1-weighted images pre and post contrast. AMH, FSH, TSH, LH, fT 4 E, PROG, PROL, TESTOST and DHEAS were measured on day 3 of the menstrual cycle before UAE. C reactive protein (CRP) and white blood cell count lab exams were carried out prior to and after UAE. Two patients that had undergone fibromyectomy and with fibromyoma recurrence were included. Preoperative imaging management enhances the ability to diagnosis and to identify pathology induced anatomic changes and is crucial in optimizing information to treatment.

Transvaginal ultrasonography (TVUS) has an efficacy of 65–99% and consists the gold standard for imaging of the woman's pelvis. MRI is crucial in the diagnosis. Differential diagnosis with MRI has a sensitivity of 88% - 93% and a specificity of 66% - 91%. MRI examination is important to rule out malignancy in the uterus, eg sarcoma and to identify nondegenerated fibroids. Degenarated fibroids occur as hyalinized fibroids, cystic changes as hypertense, myxoid degeneration as high signal intensity, necrotizing has components of necrotizing or coagulative necrosis.

9.2 UAE

All patients had signed a written consent before the UAE. The UAE procedures were performed in the hybrid angiography suite of Radiology Department using a biplane angiography system (Philips Allura Xper Cath/angio system, Koninklijke Philips N.V.).

Bilateral UAE was performed, under local anesthesia, i.v. antibiotic prophylaxis, and sedation when required. In all cases a bladder catheter has been placed.

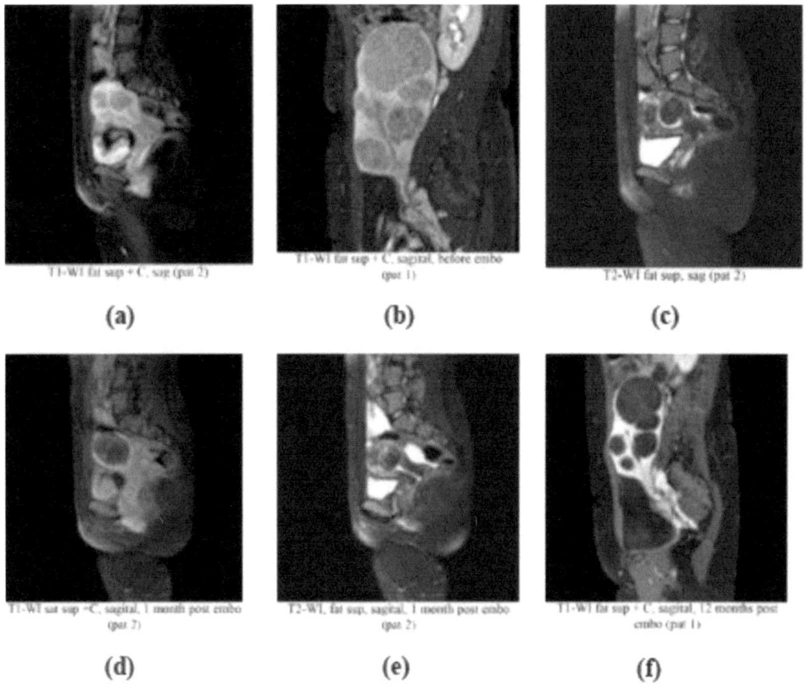

Figure 2.
MRI imaging of fibroid course pre- and post embolization.

The procedure included a single percutaneous puncture of the right common femoral artery, selective crossover contralateral and unilateral advance of a 4-French flush angiographic catheter (Simmons 1 or Cobra 1) to both uterine arteries. When the catheter bypassed the arteries for the vagina and cervix, administration of the embolic particles started. In the most of the cases a 2.7-Frence or 2.8-Frence micro-catheter (Progreat, Terumo Europe, Leuven, Belgium) has then been positioned away from the cervicovaginal branches (**Figure 2a-f**).

Special radiation protection care was taken, using fluoroscopic guidance of the catheterizations, fluoroscopy time reduction to the minimal possible and, mostly, fluoroscopic imaging of contrast angiography opacifications.

Fibroid ischemia was achieved by using of spherical, tightly calibrated, bio-compatible, non-resorbable, hydrogel coated microspheres, 700 μm and 900 μm in diameter (Embozene, CeloNova BioSciences Inc./Boston Scientific, San Antonio, USA). The angiographic embolization endpoint was defined as complete stasis of contrast agent in the ascending segment of the uterine artery during selective digital subtraction angiography at the end of the embolization procedure. Adenomyosis patients were embolized with the use of 500 μm and/or 700 μm Embozene microspheres. Criterion for the particle administration stop in adenomyosis cases was the fluoroscopic finding of "almost complete stasis".

9.3 Postprocedureal management

Regarding pain treatment, post-intervention 50 mg of pethidine was intramuscular administered, and after 4 hours the dosage was repeated by intramuscular injection in the first 24 hours. 100 mg tramadol was taken every 6 hours and anti-inflammatory tablets were taken every 12 hours for a week. Pain assessment results were determined based on a visual analogue scale (0 min-10max). After daily stay at the hospital, patients were discharged and administered broad spectrum antibiotics for one week. Clinical, laboratory and imaging follow up examinations by trans–vaginal ultrasonography and MRI scans of the patients were performed at the 1rst, 3rd, 6th and 12th month after the procedure (**Figure 1e-f**).

Main outcome measures were menstruation, hormonal status and presence of menopausal symptoms. Hormonal status and ovarian reserve were evaluated by means of AMH and FSH serum levels on 1st, 3rd, 6th and 12th month after UAE. Subsequently, FSH and LH levels began to decrease and reached the base line values on the 12th month after UAE (**Figure 3**) [71]. The AMH levels showed a decrease on the 1st month, reaching the minimum values on the 3rd month and retaining the base line values on the 3rd month in contrary to the other examined hormones. No Case of amenorrhea was noted in women ≤45 years old, while 0.6% of women >45 years old experienced amenorrhea only the first 3 months after UAE (**Figure 4**) [71] According to our findings, a leukocytosis value of up to 16,000 K/μl and an increase in CRP level of up to 8 mg/dl, are not alarming [70]. In our study were included only premenopausal women and especially women who completed their family planning. However, reported two unplanned pregnancy cases, which they have decided to terminate the pregnancy. We have no noticed no case for emergency hysterectomy. In **Table 1** are summarized the complications in our participants and according to international literature with the maximally respectively referred complications rate. The first column of the table refers to our results in the time from 2008 to 2020 while in the second column are shown the respective values of the examinated parameters in average concerning to international literature [72–76].

The course of myoma size according to a follow up for a period of 1 year post UAE was mean reduction 75% of fibroid volume compared to fibroid size before beginning of treatment. The percentage of technical success of the performed UAEs was estimated at 100% and the MRI examinations revealed that the uterine volume continues to shrink over follow up time. In no case was noticed continuity of worsening preprocedure symptoms, permanent amenorrhea, necessity of subsequent hysterectomy or minimal shrinkage of fibroid size after 6 months postprocedural. The positive results expressed as clinical included: Reduce of bleeding and pressure symptoms and as imaging reduction in uterine size and fibroids. According to our

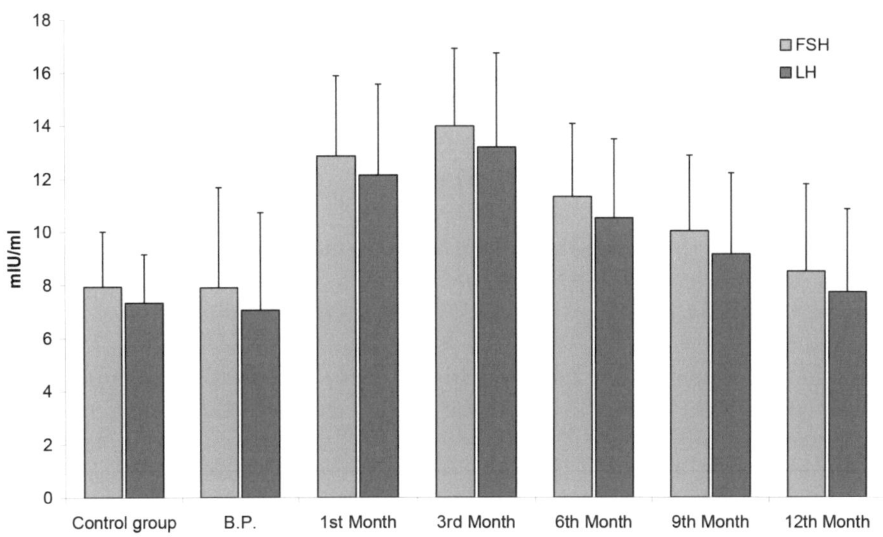

Figure 3.
Hormonal changes (FSH,LH) during the follow up period (Tsikouras et al. [71]).

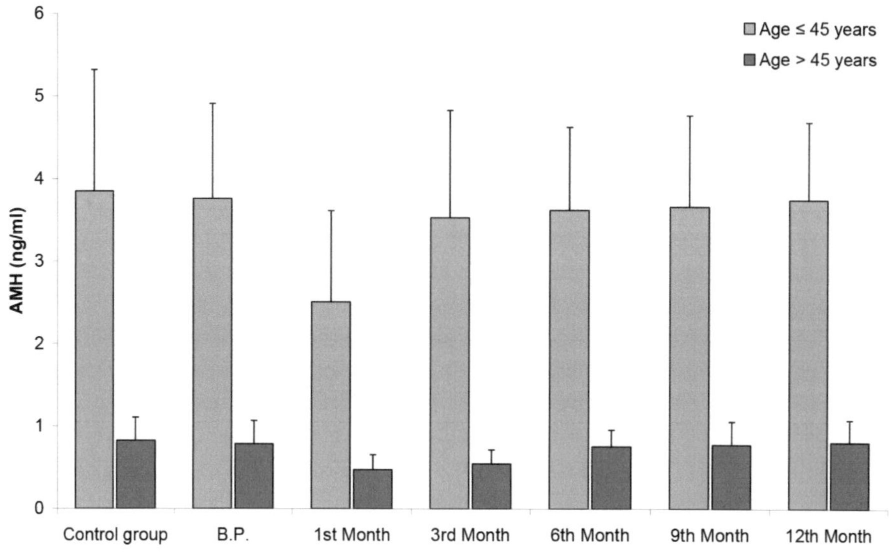

Figure 4.
Hormonal changes (AMH) during the follow up period (Tsikouras et al. [71]).

	Our results Range (min-max)	International literature results Range (min-max)
Transient amenorrhea		
< 45 years old	0.2–0.5%	1–2%
> 45 years old	1.5%	2–4%
Permanent amenorrhea	0	
< 45 years old	0	2–3%
> 45 years old	0	5–6%
Fibroma protrusion	0.3%	
Aseptic endometritis	0.1–0.2%	2%
Septic endometritis	0	1.2%
Uterine necrosis	0	<1%
Unsuccessful UAE	0	<1%

Table 1.
UAE complications: our results and various published reports.

findings after UAE the fibroids shrank by 60–70% and the size of the uterus by 50–60%. In particular, mild symptoms of metabolic syndrome in four cases were observed. Over time, shrinkage increases. The reduction in symptoms is expected to be close to 98%.

Specifically, menstruation improved in 95–100% of cases, while symptoms (flatulence, pelvic pressure and frequency) are reduced to 91–100% depending on how the result is calculated. High satisfaction rates for women. The recurrence of fibroids reaches 4%, but is thought to be due to an increase in the size of old incomplete embolized myomas and adenomyosis. The main cause of failure was not the initial size of the fibroids, but their failure shrank below 30% of the original size. In three cases it was mandatory to repeat the procedure of UAE due to the anatomical location of the fibroids, intra-ligamentally.

10. Discussion

UAE is a minimally invasive procedure which improves symptoms by interrupting the blood flow uterine vessel branches to fibroids after bilateral (from right and left) hyper-selective catheterization of the myometric feeder arteries and embossing of pistons induceing irreversible ischemic damage and degeneration/shrinkage in the fibroids [65, 75–80]. According to bibliography, therapy success rate during menorrhagia, was is 80–100% and at? pressure phenomena 60–100%. A decrease in fibroid size by 40–70% was noted in the first 6 months, followed by 50–80% in the months that ensued [67, 77–82]. There are various reports regarding uterus size course [67, 77–82]. Some authors mention uterus size as criteria, whilst others use both fibroids and uterus size as successful therapy assessment criteria. Inflammation appearance rate is 1–2% based on tissue reactions due to post interventional ischemia is an interaction between cells and cytokine and should be diagnosed at an early stage so that sepsis, hysterectomy and death can be avoided [81–84]. There have been reports of 100.000 successful UAEs in total so far [84–87].

Patients should be notified in detail and contact their doctor. Fundamental is the co-operation between gynecologist and interventional radiologist before, during and after UAE. In general, complications include either catheterization or the effects of uterine ischemia that can cause fibrotic necrosis, pain and septic imaging. The ovaries may be affected. The reported deaths following UAE are extremely rare (approximately 1: 1600) and are mainly related to pulmonary embolism, which may be due to the effect of necrotic tissue on activation of the coagulation mechanism and on inflammation. The complications of catheterization are rare (<1%), such as hematoma, allergy to contrast media and pseudo-aneurysm or vascular separation [75, 76, 87–90]. Elimination of uterine fibroids occurs in 5% of cases and can cause inflammation requiring scanning or hysterectomy. The necrotic tissue, if not removed in time, can become infected and the condition becomes severe. Cases with submucosal fibroids should be treated hysteroscopically [75, 76, 87–90]. Ischemia may cause endometritis, pelvic inflammation and pyometra with poor outcome if hysterectomy does not occur. According to the literature, menorrhagia is successfully treated in 91–100% of cases, while symptoms such as flatulence, pressure on organs of the pelvis and loss of urine are reduced to 92–100% [67, 75, 76, 87–90]. Uterine size does not appear to be a determinant, as remission of symptoms is also common in patients with a uterus greater than 24 weeks gestation. These results are also confirmed by studies of the last four years, which show that patients are 98–1000% satisfied [67, 75, 76, 87–90]. UAEs also have a beneficial effect in cases of adenomyosis, although there is not much experience. In a series of 28 patients with genuine adenomyosis an improvement of 95.3% was recorded [67, 75, 76, 87–90]. Although there are no long-term data, follow-up of up to 72 months shows postembolization syndrome include: pain and cramps (eliminated in the first hours after procedure with good/systemic analgesic treatment), nausea and fever (controlled with appropriate medications), aseptic or (rarely) septic inflammation (in a few patients, total 4 in our study controlled with anti-inflammatory/antibiotics) for 3–6 months) or (rare) menopause after UAE (small number of patients, almost always aged>45 years) [67, 75, 76, 87–90]. In these cases were diagnosed large fibroids and the reported complications affect range according to published literature 2–15% needed readmission for monitoring of symptoms. The necessity of hysterectomy after UAE approximately reported in 1% of cases. In our study participants reintervention was necessary only in 4 cases due the anatomical fibroid positions. According to international literature reintervention's rate is by 9% at 1 year and 28% at 5 years [67, 75, 76, 87–90]. Pregnancies in the majority after the UAE reported and delivered at term without serious complications, however the cesarean section rate is high approximately 33–50% [67, 75, 76, 87–91]. Based on current medical knowledge concerning genetics and molecular biology of uterine fibroids will be the basis of development microarray analysis to investigate genes, which involved in fibroid formation and provide more specific and effective minimally preventive fibroid therapies to early intervention and improve the life impact of women.

11. Conclusion

UAE is a safe and effective treatment option for uterine fibroids with international recognition, however further multicentric studies required to provide clinical data and participate in randomized control trial to compare with the known surgical procedures.

Author details

Panagiotis Tsikouras[1*], Anastasia Bothou[1], Xanthoula Anthoulaki[1], Anna Chalkidou[1], Spyridon Michalopoulos[1], Nistikoulis George[2], Ioannis Tsirkas[1], Fotini Gaitatzi[1], Selma Gyroglou[1], Irene Babageorgaka[1], Natalia Sachnova[1], Michael Koutsogiannis[1], Apostolos Lazarou[1], Arsou Chalil Bouratzan[1], Theopi Nalbanti[1], Panagiotis Peitsidis[3], Konstantinos Nikolettos[1], George Dragoutsos[1], Thedosia Vogaitzaki[4], Stefanos Zervoudis[3], George Iatrakis[3], Werner Rath[1], Nikolaos Nikolettos[1] and Vasileios Souftas[2]

1 Department of Obstetrics and Gynecology, Democritus University of Thrace, Greece

2 Department of Interventional Radiology and Medical Imaging, Democritus University of Thrace, Greece

3 Department of Obstetrics and Gynecology, Rea Hospital, Athens, Greece

4 Department of Anesthesiology, Democritus University of Thrace, Greece

*Address all correspondence to: ptsikour@med.duth.gr

References

[1] Stewart EA Uterine fibroids. Lancet. 2001 Jan 27;357 (9252):293-8 PMID:11214143 DOI: 10.1016/S0140-6736(00)03622-9

[2] Calaf J, Arqué M, Porta O, D'Angelo E The fibroid as clinical problem. Med Clin (Barc). 2013 Jul;141 Suppl 1:1-6.PMID: 24314560 DOI:10.1016/S0025-7753(13)70045-9

[3] Csatlós E, Rigó J Jr, Szabó I, Nagy Z, Joó JG.Uterine leiomyoma Orv Hetil. 2010 Oct 17;151(42):1734-41. PMID: 20889441 doi: 10.1556/OH.2010.28977. Review.

[4] .Deborah J DeWaay [1] , Craig H Syrop, Ingrid E Nygaard, William A Davis, Bradley J Van Voorhis Natural history of uterine polyps and leiomyomata Obstet Gynecol 2002 Jul;100(1):3-7. PMID: 12100797 DOI: 10.1016/s0029-7844(02)02007-0

[5] MyersER,BarberMD,Gustilo-AshbyT, Couchman G, Matchar DB, McCrory DC. Management of uterine leiomyomata: what do we really know? Obstet Gynecol. 2002 Jul;100(1):8-17. PMID: 12100798 doi: 10.1016/s0029-7844(02)02019-7. Review

[6] De La Cruz MS, Buchanan EM. Uterine Fibroids: Diagnosis and Treatment. Am Fam Physician. 2017 Jan 15;95(2):100-107. PMID: 28084714 Review

[7] O'Sullivan M, Overton C. Tailor management to the patient with fibroids Practitioner. 2017 Mar;261(1802):19-22. PMID: 29139277

[8] Vilos GA, Allaire C, Laberge PY, Leyland N; Special Contributors. The management of uterine leiomyomas. J Obstet Gynaecol Can. 2015 Feb;37(2):157-178. PMID: 25767949 doi: 10.1016/S1701-2163(15)30338-8.

[9] Payson M, Leppert P, Segars J. Epidemiology of myomas. Obstet Gynecol Clin North Am. 2006 Mar;33(1):1-11. PMID: 16504803 doi: 10.1016/j.ogc.2005.12.004.

[10] Giuliani E, As-Sanie S, Marsh EE.Epidemiology and management of uterine fibroids. Int J Gynaecol Obstet. 2020 Apr;149(1):3-9. doi: 10.1002/ijgo.13102. Epub 2020 Feb 17. PMID: 31960950 Review

[11] Okolo S. Incidence, aetiology and epidemiology of uterine fibroids. Best Pract Res Clin Obstet Gynaecol. 2008 Aug;22(4):571-88. doi: 10.1016/j.bpobgyn.2008.04.002. Epub 2008 Jun 4. PMID: 18534913 Review

[12] Baird DD, et al. High cumulative incidence of uterine leiomyoma in black and white women: ultrasound evidence. Am J Obstet Gynecol. 2003. PMID: 12548202

[13] Wise LA, Palmer JR, Stewart EA, Rosenberg L. Age-specific incidence rates for self-reported uterine leiomyomata in the Black Women's Health Study. Obstet Gynecol. 2005 Mar;105(3):563-8. PMID: 15738025 doi: 10.1097/01.AOG.0000154161.03418.e3.

[14] Baird DD, et al. Why is parity protective for uterine fibroids? Epidemiology. 2003. PMID: 12606893

[15] Heinemann K, Thiel C, Möhner S, Lewis MA, Raff T, Kühl-Habich D, Heinemann LA; Benign gynecological tumors: estimated incidence. Results of the German Cohort Study on Women's Health. German Cohort Study on Women's Health. Eur J Obstet Gynecol Reprod Biol. 2003 Mar 26;107(1):78-80. doi: 10.1016/s0301-2115(02)00308-1. PMID: 12593900

[16] Wise LA, Palmer JR, Harlow BL, Spiegelman D, Stewart EA,

Adams-Campbell LL, Rosenberg L Reproductive factors, hormonal contraception, and risk of uterine leiomyomata in African-American women: a prospective study. Am J Epidemiol. 2004 Jan 15;159(2):113-23. doi: 10.1093/aje/kwh016. PMID: 14718211

[17] .Radosa MP, Owsianowski Z, Mothes A, Weisheit A, Vorwergk J, Asskaryar FA, Camara O, Bernardi TS, Runnebaum IB. Long-term risk of fibroid recurrence after laparoscopic myomectomy. Eur J Obstet Gynecol Reprod Biol. 2014 Sep;180:35-9.. PMID: 25016181 doi: 10.1016/j.ejogrb.2014.05.029. Epub 2014 Jun 2

[18] Horng HC, Wen KC, Su WH, Chen CS, Wang PH. Review of myomectomy. Taiwan J Obstet Gynecol. 2012 Mar;51(1):7-11. PMID: 22482961 Review. doi: 10.1016/j.tjog.2012.01.003.

[19] Jacoby VL, Fujimoto VY, Giudice LC, Kuppermann M, Washington AE Racial and ethnic disparities in benign gynecologic conditions and associated surgeries. Am J Obstet Gynecol. 2010 Jun;202(6):514-21. doi: 10.1016/j.ajog.2010.02.039. Epub 2010 Apr 28. PMID: 20430357

[20] Laughlin-Tommaso SK, Jacoby VL, Myers ER. Disparities in Fibroid Incidence, Prognosis, and Management. Obstet Gynecol Clin North Am. 2017 Mar;44(1):81-94. PMID: 28160895 doi: 10.1016/j.ogc.2016.11.007.

[21] Melissa K Lobel , Priya Somasundaram, Cynthia C Morton The genetic heterogeneity of uterine leiomyomata Obstet Gynecol Clin North Am 2006 Mar;33(1):13-39. PMID: 16504804 DOI: 10.1016/j.ogc.2005.12.006

[22] . Luoto R, Kaprio J, Rutanen EM, Taipale P, Perola M, Koskenvuo M Heritability and risk factors of uterine fibroids--the Finnish Twin Cohort study. Maturitas. 2000 Nov 30;37(1):15-26. doi: 10.1016/s0378-5122(00)00160-2. PMID: 11099869

[23] Sandberg AA. Updates on the cytogenetics and molecular genetics of bone and soft tissue tumors: leiomyoma.

[24] Laganà AS, Vergara D, Favilli A, La Rosa VL, Tinelli A, Gerli S, Noventa M, Vitagliano A, Triolo O, Rapisarda AMC, Vitale SG. Epigenetic and genetic landscape of uterine leiomyomas: a current view over a common gynecological disease. Arch Gynecol Obstet. 2017 Nov;296(5):855-867. doi: 10.1007/s00404-017-4515-5. Epub 2017 Sep 5. PMID: 28875276 Review.

[25] Catherino W, Salama A, Potlog-Nahari C, Leppert P, Tsibris J, Segars J. Semin Gene expression studies in leiomyomata: new directions for research. Reprod Med. 2004 May;22(2):83-90. doi: 10.1055/s-2004-828614. PMID: 15164303 Review.

[26] Ligon AH, Morton CC. Genetics of uterine leiomyomata. Genes Chromosomes Cancer. 2000 Jul;28(3):235-45. PMID: 10862029 Review.

[27] Flake GP, Andersen J, Dixon D. Etiology and pathogenesis of uterine leiomyomas: a review. Environ Health Perspect. 2003 Jun;111(8):1037-54. doi: 10.1289/ehp.5787. PMID: 12826476

[28] Segars JH, Parrott EC, Nagel JD, Guo XC, Gao X, Birnbaum LS, Pinn VW, Dixon D. Proceedings from the Third National Institutes of Health International Congress on Advances in Uterine Leiomyoma Research: comprehensive review, conference summary and future recommendations. Hum Reprod Update. 2014 May-Jun;20(3):309-33. doi: 10.1093/humupd/dmt058. Epub 2014 Jan 8. PMID: 24401287

[29] Avery A Sandberg Updates on the cytogenetics and molecular genetics of bone and soft tissue tumors: leiomyoma Cancer Genet Cytogenet. 2005 Apr 1;158(1):1-26. doi: 10.1016/j.cancergencyto.2004.08.025. PMID: 15771900 Review.

[30] Ishwad CS, Ferrell RE, Davare J, Meloni AM, Sandberg AA, Surti U Molecular and cytogenetic analysis of chromosome 7 in uterine leiomyomas. Genes Chromosomes Cancer. 1995 Sep;14(1):51-5. doi: 10.1002/gcc.2870140109. PMID: 8527384

[31] Erica E Marsh, Zhihong Lin, Ping Yin, Magdy Milad, Debabrata Chakravarti, Serdar E Bulun Differential expression of microRNA species in human uterine leiomyoma versus normal myometrium Fertil Steril 2008 Jun;89(6):1771-6. PMID: 17765232 DOI:10.1016/j.fertnstert.2007.05.074

[32] Karmon AE, Cardozo ER, Rueda BR, Styer AK. MicroRNAs in the development and pathobiology of uterine leiomyomata: does evidence support future strategies for clinical intervention? Hum Reprod Update. 2014 Sep-Oct;20(5):670-87. doi: 10.1093/humupd/dmu017. Epub 2014 Apr 4. PMID: 24706045 Review.

[33] Wei MH, Toure O, Glenn GM, Pithukpakorn M, Neckers L, Stolle C, Choyke P, Grubb R, Middelton L, Turner ML, Walther MM, Merino MJ, Zbar B, Linehan WM, Toro JR. Novel mutations in FH and expansion of the spectrum of phenotypes expressed in families with hereditary leiomyomatosis and renal cell cancer. J Med Genet. 2006 Jan;43(1):18-27. doi: 10.1136/jmg.2005.033506. Epub 2005 Jun 3. PMID: 15937070

[34] Fejzo MS, Yoon SJ, Montgomery KT, Rein MS, Weremowicz S, Krauter KS, Dorman TE, Fletcher JA, Mao JI, Moir DT, et al. Identification of a YAC spanning the translocation breakpoints in uterine leiomyomata, pulmonary chondroid hamartoma, and lipoma: physical mapping of the 12q14-q15 breakpoint region in uterine leiomyomata. Genomics. 1995 Mar 20;26(2):265-71. doi: 10.1016/0888-7543(95)80210-d. PMID: 7601452

[35] Lohle PNM, Higué D, Herbreteau D. Uterine artery embolisation in women with symptomatic adenomyosis. Presse Med. 2019 Apr;48(4):435-439. doi: 10.1016/j.lpm.2019.03.013. Epub 2019 Apr 27. PMID: 31036387

[36] Bruce McLucas, Rita Perrella Adenomyosis: MRI of the uterus treated with uterine artery embolization AJR Am J Roentgenol 2004 Apr;182(4):1084-5; author reply 1085. PMID: 15039193 doi: 10.2214/ajr.182.4.1821084a.

[37] Jha RC, Takahama J, Imaoka I, Korangy SJ, Spies JB, Cooper C, Ascher SM. Adenomyosis: MRI of the uterus treated with uterine artery embolization. AJR Am J Roentgenol. 2003 Sep;181(3):851-6. doi: 10.2214/ajr.181.3.1810851. PMID: 12933493

[38] Dundr P, Mára M, Masková J, Fucíková Z, Povỳsil C, Tvrdík D. Pathological findings of uterine leiomyomas and adenomyosis following uterine artery embolization. Pathol Res Pract. 2006;202(10):721-9. doi: 10.1016/j.prp.2006.07.001. Epub 2006 Sep 7. PMID: 16959435

[39] Rabinovici J, Stewart EA. New interventional techniques for adenomyosis. Best Pract Res Clin Obstet Gynaecol. 2006 Aug;20(4):617-36. doi: 10.1016/j.bpobgyn.2006.02.002. Epub 2006 Aug 24. PMID: 16934530

[40] Kitamura Y Allison SJ, Jha RC, Spies JB, Flick PA, Ascher SM.MRI of adenomyosis: changes with uterine artery embolization.AJR Am J Roentgenol. 2006 Mar;186(3):855-64.

[41] Kim MD, Kim S, Kim NK, Lee MH, Ahn EH, Kim HJ, Cho JH, Cha SH. Long-term results of uterine artery embolization for symptomatic adenomyosis.AJR Am J Roentgenol. 2007 Jan;188(1):176-81.

[42] Gordts S, Grimbizis G, Campo R Symptoms and classification of uterine adenomyosis, including the place of hysteroscopy in diagnosis.. Fertil Steril. 2018 Mar;109(3):380-388.e1. doi: 10.1016/j.fertnstert.2018.01.006. PMID: 29566850 Review.

[43] Bukulmez O, Doody KJ. Clinical features of myomas. Obstet Gynecol Clin North Am. 2006 Mar;33(1):69-84. doi: 10.1016/j.ogc.2005.12.002. PMID: 16504807

[44] Gupta S, Jose J, Manyonda I. Clinical presentation of fibroids. Best Pract Res Clin Obstet Gynaecol. 2008 Aug;22(4):615-26. doi: 10.1016/j.bpobgyn.2008.01.008. Epub 2008 Mar 26. PMID: 18372219 Review.

[45] Angioni S, Loddo A, Milano F, Piras B, Minerba L, Melis GB.Detection of benign intracavitary lesions in postmenopausal women with abnormal uterine bleeding: a prospective comparative study on outpatient hysteroscopy and blind biopsy. J Minim Invasive Gynecol. 2008 Jan-Feb;15(1):87-91. doi: 10.1016/j.jmig.2007.10.014. PMID: 18262151

[46] Russo M, Suen M, Bedaiwy M, Chen I. Prevalence of Uterine Myomas Among Women with 2 or More Recurrent Pregnancy Losses: A Systematic Review. J Minim Invasive Gynecol. 2016 Jul-Aug;23(5):702-6. doi:10.1016/j.jmig.2016.03.018. Epub 2016 Mar 31. PMID: 27041652 Review.

[47] Wallach EE, Vlahos NF.Uterine myomas: an overview of development, clinical features, and management. Obstet Gynecol. 2004 Aug;104(2):393-406. doi: 10.1097/01.AOG.0000136079.62513.39. PMID: 15292018 Review.

[48] Kjerulff KH, Langenberg P, Seidman JD, Stolley PD, Guzinski GM. Uterine leiomyomas. Racial differences in severity, symptoms and age at diagnosis. J Reprod Med. 1996 Jul;41(7):483-90. PMID: 8829060

[49] Stovall DW Clinical symptomatology of uterine leiomyomas. Clin Obstet Gynecol. 2001 Jun;44(2):364-71. doi: 10.1097/00003081-200106000-00022. PMID: 11344999 Review.

[50] Leung F, Terzibachian JJ, Gay C, Chung Fat B, Aouar Z, Lassabe C, Maillet R, Riethmuller D. Hysterectomies performed for presumed leiomyomas: should the fear of leiomyosarcoma make us apprehend non laparotomic surgical routes?. Gynecol Obstet Fertil. 2009 Feb;37(2):109-14. doi: 10.1016/j.gyobfe.2008.09.022. Epub 2009 Feb 5. PMID: 19200764

[51] Rackow BW, Arici A Options for medical treatment of myomas. Obstet Gynecol Clin North Am. 2006 Mar;33(1):97-113. doi: 10.1016/j.ogc.2005.12.014. PMID: 16504809 Review.

[52] Donnez J, Courtoy GE, Dolmans MM. Fibroid management in premenopausal women. Climacteric. 2019 Feb;22(1):27-33. doi: 10.1080/13697137.2018.1549216. Epub 2019 Jan 2. PMID: 30601065

[53] Donnez J, Dolmans MM. Uterine fibroid management: from the present to the future. Hum Reprod Update. 2016 Nov;22(6):665-686. doi: 10.1093/humupd/dmw023. Epub 2016 Jul 27. PMID: 27466209

[54] Lethaby A, Vollenhoven B, Sowter M. Efficacy of pre-operative gonadotrophin hormone releasing analogues for women with uterine

fibroids undergoing hysterectomy or myomectomy: a systematic review. BJOG. 2002 Oct;109(10):1097-108. doi: 10.1111/j.1471-0528.2002.01225.x. PMID: 12387461

[55] Lethaby A, Vollenhoven B, Sowter M. Pre-operative GnRH analogue therapy before hysterectomy or myomectomy for uterine fibroids. Cochrane Database Syst Rev. 2001;(2):CD000547. doi: 10.1002/14651858.CD000547. PMID: 11405968

[56] Lethaby A, Puscasiu L, Vollenhoven B. Preoperative medical therapy before surgery for uterine fibroids. Cochrane Database Syst Rev. 2017 Nov 15;11(11):CD000547. doi: 10.1002/14651858.CD000547.pub2. PMID: 29139105

[57] Sankaran S, Manyonda IT. Medical management of fibroids. Best Pract Res Clin Obstet Gynaecol. 2008 Aug;22(4):655-76. doi: 10.1016/j.bpobgyn.2008.03.001. Epub 2008 May 12. PMID: 18468953 Review.

[58] Islam MS, Protic O, Giannubilo SR, Toti P, Tranquilli AL, Petraglia F, Castellucci M, Ciarmela P. Uterine leiomyoma: available medical treatments and new possible therapeutic options. J Clin Endocrinol Metab. 2013 Mar;98(3):921-34. doi: 10.1210/jc.2012-3237. Epub 2013 Feb 7. PMID: 23393173 Review.

[59] Lethaby AE, Vollenhoven BJ. An evidence-based approach to hormonal therapies for premenopausal women with fibroids. Best Pract Res Clin Obstet Gynaecol. 2008 Apr;22(2): 307-31. doi: 10.1016/j.bpobgyn.2007.07.010. Epub 2007 Oct 1. PMID: 17905660 Review.

[60] Bouchard P, Ouzounian S, Chabbert-Buffet N. Selective progesterone receptor modulators: future clinical applications. Bull Acad Natl Med. 2008 Jun-Jul;192(6):1159-71; discussion 1172-3. PMID: 19235480

[61] Laberge PY, Murji A, Vilos GA, Allaire C, Leyland N, Singh SS. Guideline No. 389-Medical Management of Symptomatic Uterine Leiomyomas - An Addendum. J Obstet Gynaecol Can. 2019 Oct;41(10):1521-1524. doi: 10.1016/j.jogc.2019.01.010. PMID: 3154804

[62] Elahi SM, Odejinmi F Overview of current surgical management of fibroids: 'Organ-preserving modalities'. J Obstet Gynaecol. 2008 Jan;28(1):28-31. doi: 10.1080/01443610701814328. PMID: 18259894 Review.

[63] Liu WM, Wang PH, Chou CS, Tang WL, Wang IT, Tzeng CR. Efficacy of combined laparoscopic uterine artery occlusion and myomectomy via minilaparotomy in the treatment of recurrent uterine myomas. Fertil Steril. 2007 Feb;87(2):356-61. doi: 10.1016/j.fertnstert.2006.07.1497. Epub 2006 Oct 25. PMID: 17069812 Clinical Trial.

[64] Kaminski P, Gajewska M, Wielgos M, Sodowski K, Szymusik I, Bartkowiak R, Marianowski P, Czuba B. Laparoscopic treatment of uterine myomas in women of reproductive age. Neuro Endocrinol Lett. 2008 Feb;29(1):163-7. PMID: 18283255

[65] Agdi M, Tulandi T Endoscopic management of uterine fibroids. Best Pract Res Clin Obstet Gynaecol. 2008 Aug;22(4):707-16. doi: 10.1016/j.bpobgyn.2008.01.011. Epub 2008 Mar 6. PMID: 18325839 Review.

[66] Keserci B, Duc NM, Nadarajan C, Huy HQ, Saizan A, Wan Ahmed WA, Osman K, Abdullah MS. Volumetric MRI-guided, high-intensity focused ultrasound ablation of uterine leiomyomas: ASEAN preliminary experience. Diagn Interv Radiol. 2020 May;26(3):207-215. doi: 10.5152/dir.2019.19157. PMID: 32209511

[67] Marshburn PB, Matthews ML, Hurst BS. Uterine artery embolization as a treatment option for uterine myomas. Obstet Gynecol Clin North Am. 2006 Mar;33(1):125-44. doi: 10.1016/j.ogc.2005.12.009. PMID: 16504811 Review.

[68] Zurawin RK, Fischer JH 2nd, Amir L The effect of a gynecologist-interventional radiologist relationship on selection of treatment modality for the patient with uterine myoma. J Minim Invasive Gynecol. 2010 Mar-Apr;17(2):214-21. doi: 10.1016/j.jmig.2009.12.015. PMID: 20226411

[69] Istre O. Management of symptomatic fibroids: conservative surgical treatment modalities other than abdominal or laparoscopic myomectomy. Best Pract Res Clin Obstet Gynaecol. 2008 Aug;22(4):735-47. doi: 10.1016/j.bpobgyn.2008.01.010. Epub 2008 Mar 7. PMID: 18328788 Review

[70] Lupattelli T, Clerissi J, Basile A, Minnella DP, Donati Sarti R, Gerli S, Di Renzo G. Treatment of uterine fibromyoma with bilateral uterine artery embolization: state of the art. Minerva Ginecol. 2007 Aug;59(4):427-39. PMID: 17923833 Review.

[71] Tsikouras P, Manav B, Koukouli Z, Trypsiannis G, Galazios G, Souftas D, Souftas V. Ovarian reserve after fibroid embolization in premenopausal women. Minim Invasive Ther Allied Technol. 2017 Oct;26(5):284-291. doi: 10.1080/13645706.2017.1292919. Epub 2017 Feb 24. PMID: 28635407

[72] Souftas V, Deuteraiou D, Anthoulaki X, Chalkidou A, Bothou A, Gaidatzi F, Tsypsianis G, Iatrakis G, Zervoudis S, Souftas D, Michalopoulos S, Vogiatzaki T, Galazios G, Nikolettos N, Tsikouras P. Significance of changes in inflammatory parameters following uterine artery embolization in pre-menopausal females. Exp Ther Med. 2020 Jun;19(6):3684-3690. doi: 10.3892/etm.2020.8652. Epub 2020 Apr 9. PMID: 32346432

[73] Armstrong AA, Kroener L, Brower M, Al-Safi ZA. Analysis of Reported Adverse Events with Uterine Artery Embolization for Leiomyomas. J Minim Invasive Gynecol. 2019 May-Jun;26(4):667-670.e1. doi: 10.1016/j.jmig.2018.07.006. Epub 2018 Aug 29. PMID: 30016750

[74] Soeda S, Hiraiwa T, Takata M, Kamo N, Sekino H, Nomura S, Kojima M, Kyozuka H, Ozeki T, Ishii S, Tameda T, Asano K, Miyazaki M, Takahashi T, Watanabe T, Taki Y, Fujimori K. Unique Learning System for Uterine Artery Embolization for Symptomatic Myoma and Adenomyosis for Obstetrician-Gynecologists in Cooperation with Interventional Radiologists: Evaluation of UAE From the Point of View of Gynecologists Who Perform UAE. J Minim Invasive Gynecol. 2018 Jan;25(1):84-92. doi: 10.1016/j.jmig.2017.08.008. Epub 2017 Aug 12. PMID: 28807810

[75] Mutiso SK, Oindi FM, Hacking N, Obura T. Uterine Necrosis after Uterine Artery Embolization for Symptomatic Fibroids. Case Rep Obstet Gynecol. 2018 May 28;2018:9621741. doi: 10.1155/2018/9621741. eCollection 2018. PMID: 29998027

[76] Toor SS, Jaberi A, Macdonald DB, McInnes MD, Schweitzer ME, Rasuli P. Complication rates and effectiveness of uterine artery embolization in the treatment of symptomatic leiomyomas: a systematic review and meta-analysis. AJR Am J Roentgenol. 2012 Nov;199(5):1153-63. doi: 10.2214/AJR.11.8362. PMID: 23096193

[77] Olive DL, Lindheim SR, Pritts EA Conservative surgical management of uterine myomas. Obstet Gynecol Clin North Am. 2006 Mar;33(1):115-24. doi: 10.1016/j.ogc.2005.12.012. PMID: 16504810

[78] Marret H, Fritel X, Ouldamer L, Bendifallah S, Brun JL, De Jesus I, Derrien J, Giraudet G, Kahn V, Koskas M, Legendre G, Lucot JP, Niro J, Panel P, Pelage JP, Fernandez H; CNGOF (French College of Gynecology and Obstetrics). Therapeutic management of uterine fibroid tumors: updated French guidelines. Eur J Obstet Gynecol Reprod Biol. 2012 Dec;165(2):156-64. doi: 10.1016/j.ejogrb.2012.07.030. Epub 2012 Aug 29. PMID: 22939241 Review.

[79] Kalina I, Tóth A, Valcseva É, Kaposi PN, Ács N, Várbíró S, Bérczi V. Prognostic value of pre-embolisation MRI features of uterine fibroids in uterine artery embolisation. Clin Radiol. 2018 Dec;73(12):1060.e1-1060.e7. doi: 10.1016/j.crad.2018.08.009. Epub 2018 Oct 9. PMID: 30309632

[80] Katsumori T, Asai S, Yokota H, Miura H. Volume of embolic agents in uterine artery embolization for leiomyoma: relation to baseline MRI. Minim Invasive Ther Allied Technol. 2019 Jun;28(3):186-193. doi: 10.1080/13645706.2018.1513408. Epub 2018 Sep 27. PMID: 30261778

[81] Kohi MP, Spies JB. Updates on Uterine Artery Embolization. Semin Intervent Radiol. 2018 Mar;35(1):48-55. doi: 10.1055/s-0038-1636521. Epub 2018 Apr 5. PMID: 29628616

[82] Chung YJ, Kang SY, Chun HJ, Rha SE, Cho HH, Kim JH, Kim MR. Development of a Model for the Prediction of Treatment Response of Uterine Leiomyomas after Uterine Artery Embolization.Int J Med Sci. 2018 Nov 23;15(14):1771-1777. doi: 10.7150/ijms.28687. eCollection 2018.

[83] SOGC clinical practice guidelines. Uterine fibroid embolization (UFE). Number 150, October 2004. Society of Obstetricians and Gynaecologists of Canada. Int J Gynaecol Obstet. 2005 Jun;89(3):305-18. doi: 10.1016/j.ijgo.2005.03.013. PMID: 16001461 Review.

[84] Kröncke T, David M. Uterine Artery Embolization (UAE) for Fibroid Treatment - Results of the 7th Radiological Gynecological Expert Meeting. Rofo. 2019 Jul;191(7):630-634. doi: 10.1055/a-0884-3168. Epub 2019 May 28. PMID: 31137043

[85] Lohle PNM, Higué D, Herbreteau D.Uterine artery embolisation in women with symptomatic uterine fibroids. Presse Med. 2019 Apr;48(4):440-446. doi: 10.1016/j.lpm.2019.03.012. Epub 2019 Apr 27. PMID: 31036388

[86] Davis MR, Soliman AM, Castelli-Haley J, Snabes MC, Surrey ES Reintervention Rates After Myomectomy, Endometrial Ablation, and Uterine Artery Embolization for Patients with Uterine Fibroids. J Womens Health (Larchmt). 2018 Oct;27(10):1204-1214. doi: 10.1089/jwh.2017.6752. Epub 2018 Aug 7. PMID: 30085898

[87] Stępniak A.Uterine artery embolization in the treatment of symptomatic fibroids - state of the art 2018. Prz Menopauzalny. 2018 Dec;17(4):141-143. doi: 10.5114/pm.2018.81733. Epub 2018 Dec 31. PMID: 30766459

[88] El Shamy T, Amer SAK, Mohamed AA, James C, Jayaprakasan K. The impact of uterine artery embolization on ovarian reserve: A systematic review and meta-analysis. Acta Obstet Gynecol Scand. 2020 Jan;99(1):16-23. doi: 10.1111/aogs.13698. Epub 2019 Aug 26. PMID: 31370100

[89] Lacayo EA, Khera SS, Spies JB. Impact of Patient and Procedure-Related Factors on Radiation Exposure from Uterine Artery Embolization. Cardiovasc Intervent Radiol. 2020 Jan;43(1):120-126. doi: 10.1007/

s00270-019-02321-7. Epub 2019 Sep 11. PMID: 31511962

[90] Siskin GP. Optimizing Fibroid Infarction Rates after Uterine Artery Embolization. J Vasc Interv Radiol. 2019 May;30(5):677-678. doi: 10.1016/j.jvir.2018.11.040. PMID: 31029386

[91] Peitsidis P, Chernev A, Peitsidou A, Tsekoura V, Zervoudis S, Navrozoglou I, et al. Treatment of leiomyomas with uterine artery embolization. Review of literature. Bulgarian: Akush Ginekol (Sofiia); 2008;**47**(1):38-42. PMID: 18642577

Chapter 7

Physiopathology and Management of Uterine Fibroids

Joel Noutakdie Tochie, Gaelle Therese Badjang, Gregory Ayissi and Julius Sama Dohbit

Abstract

Uterine fibroid is the most encountered benign tumour in women of reproductive age. It causes spontaneous abortions, missed abortions, painful red degeneration or infarction of the fibroids, abnormal foetal presentation, obstructed labour, and an increased likelihood of premature deliveries, caesarean deliveries, postpartum haemorrhage in pregnancy, whereas, in the non-pregnant women it is associated an irregular menstrual cycle sometimes associated with heavy menstrual bleeding, infertility, constipation, urinary incontinence, and leiosarcoma transformation. Till date is pathophysiology and management both in the non-pregnant and pregnant woman have not been well described. In this chapter, we present contemporary evidence to help elucidate this enigma.

Keywords: uterine fibroid, leiomyoma, pathophysiology, management

1. Introduction

Leiomyomas also called uterine myomas, uterine fibroids, or fibromyomas are discrete, rounded, firm, white to pale pink, benign myometrial tumours composed mostly of smooth muscle with varying amounts of fibrous connective tissues [1]. Uterine fibroids or leiomyomas are benign tumours of the uterine smooth muscles. They are benign clonal neoplasms that contain an increased amount of extracellular collagen, elastin and are surrounded by a thin pseudo-capsule. They may enlarge to cause significant distortion of the uterine surface or cavity. Their size will then be described in menstrual weeks, as in a pregnant uterus [2].

Most fibroids are asymptomatic; usually asymptomatic in pregnancy but may interfere with conception and may cause spontaneous abortion, missed abortions, painful red degeneration or infarction of the fibroids, abnormal foetal presentation, obstructed labour, and an increased likelihood of premature deliveries, caesarean deliveries, postpartum haemorrhage and, whereas, in the non-pregnant state its signs and symptoms are menorrhagia, metorrhagia, menometorrhagia, infertility, constipation, urinary incontinence, and leiosarcoma transformation [3]. Uterine fibroids can occur in the non-pregnant woman and then continue into pregnancy/may develop de novo in pregnancy. In both circumstances, the physiopathology is the same but specific considerations may be taken in its management.

2. Epidemiology

Evidence from the contemporary literature reports that the prevalence rate of uterine fibroid varies between 16.7% - 30% of reproductive-age women and there is a two-fold increase in the prevalence in Afro American women [4, 5]. Also, their incidence tends to peak at the age of 35 years and almost 50% of African women will have uterine fibroid by their 5th decade of life [1]. Leiomyomas are the most frequent pelvic tumours and occur in about 20 to 25% of reproductive-age women. Uterine fibroids and the severity of their symptoms have a predilection for the black ethnicity. Huyck KL et al. in 2008 demonstrated that the odds of having severe symptoms from uterine fibroids are more than five times greater in black African women than in Caucasians [6]. Furthermore, black women develop the disease five to six years earlier and their peak age at diagnosis is 40–44 years [7] as opposed to a to peak age of incidence of 35 years observed in Caucasians [1]. Also, almost 50% of African women will have uterine fibroid by their 5th decade of life [1].

Risks factors of uterine fibroids include African-American ethnicity, early menarche (less than 11 years) and high body mass index [8, 9]. Moreover, the length of the menstrual cycle has an inversely proportional relationship with fibroids: a shorter cycle is positively correlated with an increased likelihood to develop fibroids [10, 11]. A similar inverse association is observed with use of oral contraceptives, the duration of tobacco smoking and the development of fibroids [12]. On the other hand, multiparity and the late ages of last pregnancy are other protective factors for uterine fibroids [11].

3. Anatomical Classification of Uterine Fibroids

According to their anatomic locations, there are three different types of leiomyomas:

- **Subserosal or subperitoneal** leiomyomata are the most common and are usually asymptomatic unless very large. They originate in the myometrium and grow out toward the serosal surface of the uterus, lying beneath the peritoneum [1]. They may lie just at the serosal surface of the uterus or may become pedunculated. They become parasitic when they derive their entire blood supply outside of the uterus, from omental vessels. Sometimes, their pedicles may atrophy and resorb. When they arise laterally, subserous tumours may extend between the two peritoneal layers of the broad ligament to become intraligamentary leiomyomas.

- **Intramural or interstitial** myomas are located within the uterine wall of the myometrium and may distort the shape of the uterine cavity and surface. They may manifest with swelling of the abdomen, menorrhagia and infertility.

- **Submucosal fibroids** are the most symptomatic. They originate in the myometrium and grow toward the endometrial cavity, protruding into the uterine cavity that they tend to compress. Their impact on the endometrium and its blood supply most often lead to irregular uterine bleeding. Other symptoms commonly associated are dysmenorrhea, infertility and recurrent abortions [13]. This type of fibroids may also develop pedicles and protrude fully into the uterine cavity. Occasionally they pass through the cervical canal while still attached within the corpus by a long stalk. There, they are subject to torsion or infection.

- **Cervical leiomyomas** are a rare type. They are sometimes mistaken to vaginal leiomyomas, which may present with the same clinical features [14]. They cause early pressure effects in regions of bladder neck, infection, dyspareunia and infertility.

- With respect to the location of the fibroids, 89.4% submucous, 10.6% subserous and 74.5% were intramural according to a study done in Cameroon [15].

FIGO classification of uterine fibroids (PALM-COEIN)

Stage 0: a sub-mucosal pedunculated intra-uterine cavity fibroid
Stage 1: a sub-mucosal located less than 50% intra-murally
Stage 2: a sub-mucosal located greater than 50% intra-murally
Stage 3: a fibroid which is 100% interstitially or intra-murally located in contact with the endometrium
Stage 4: a fibroid which is completely interstitially or intra-murally located
Stage 5: a sub-serosal fibroid which is greater than or equall to 50% intra-murally located
Stage 6: a sub-serosal fibroid which is less than 50% intra-murally located
Stage 7: a sub-serosal pedunculated fibroid
Stage 8: others, parasite (round cervical ligament, large ligament).

4. Physiopathology of Uterine Fibroids

The cause of uterine leiomyomata is idiopathic till date. However, several hypotheses have been postulated, namely:

i. Glucose-6-phosphate dehydrogenase studies suggest that each individual leiomyoma is unicellular in origin that is monoclonal [2]. Hence, this implies a genetic probability for the growth of uterine.

ii. In increment in the exposure of circulating oestrogens is another hypothesis for the growth of uterine fibroids. Effectively, leiomyomas contain oestrogen receptors in higher concentrations than the surrounding myometrium. But at lower concentrations than the endometrium, this oestrogen may contribute to tumour enlargement by increasing the production of extracellular matrix. On the other hand, progesterone increases the mitotic activity of myomas in young women. It may allow for tumour enlargement by down-regulating apoptosis in the fibroids [16]. They usually decrease in size after menopause and whenever myomas grow after menopause, malignancy must be seriously considered [17].

Malignant transformation of leiomyomas is very rare, seen in 0.04% women having uterine fibroids. In a review of 13,000 leiomyomas, 38 cases (0.29%) demonstrated malignant manifestations. A second study reported that malignant change developed in less than 0.13% of uterine leiomyomas [17]. The diagnosis of leiomyosarcomas is based on the counts of 10 or more mitotic figures per 10 HPFs. Atypical leiomyoma is differentiated from leiomyosarcoma by a lack of necrotizing tumour cells and a mitotic count less than 7 per 10 HPFs. Nuclear atypia makes the difference with mitotically active leiomyoma [18]. Secondary changes may occur when the fibroids tend to outgrow their blood supply. These degenerations include necrotic, haemorrhagic (red degeneration) or septic for the acute ones. Chronic degeneration may be atrophic, hyaline (65%), cystic, calcific (10%), myxomatous (15%), or fatty [1].

5. Diagnoses

5.1 Clinical features

Most at times, leiomyomas are asymptomatic. Symptoms are found only in about 35–50% of the patients. They vary according to the type, location, size, number and vascular supply of the fibroids. These include:

- Abnormal bleeding from the uterus
- Pain symptoms
- Pressure effects
- Reproductive dysfunction

Bleeding from the uterus is the most common symptom. It may either be during the menstrual periods when the patient will have heavy and prolonged menses called menometorrhagia [16] or it may manifest as light spotting before and after the menses. The incidence of abnormal uterine bleeding was 47.7% in a study done by Okogbo et al. in 2011 in Nigeria [19]. This abnormal bleeding is due to the development or dilatation of endometrial venules which increase the flow during cyclical sloughing or to the increase in size of the uterine cavity by the fibromyomas [17].

Pain may either be due to red degeneration, infarction or torsion of a uterine fibroid, or mat stem from attempts to expel a pedunculated submucousal fibroid [1]. A sensation of pelvic heaviness or fullness or a feeling of a mass in the pelvis is particularly characteristic of large tumours. These may press on nerves within the bony pelvis, creating pain that radiates to the back or lower extremities.

Pressure effects may either be anteriorly on the bladder, causing mainly frequent micturation, and urinary incontinence. Laterally, myomas may compress the ureters, leading to hydroureters. When the base of the bladder is involved, urinary retention may occur. Posteriorly, fibroids may increase the rectal pressure or cause constipation or tenesmus. It should be noted that these pressure symptoms are quite unusual and are difficult to directly relate to fibroids.

The relationship between fibroids and **infertility** is not clear. Fibroids may have a detrimental effect on fertility in up to 10% of the cases [20]. Infertility may result because of impaired implantation, tubal function or sperm transport.

5.2 Diagnostic tests

The diagnosis of uterine fibroids is made from the signs and symptoms, pelvic examination, laboratory investigations and imaging.

Most leiomyomas are discovered by routine pelvic examination, when a firm mass of an irregular shape is felt in the uterus. To confirm the diagnosis different types of imaging techniques are used:

- **A Pelvic ultrasound scan** is the test of first choice. Here, three-dimensional scan is preferred to a two-dimensional scan due its higher resolution which helps to rule out a pregnancy, other pelvic masses, a congenital uterine malformation [21].

- **A magnetic resonance imaging** is the gold standard test which is highly accurate in depicting the size, number and location of myomas to choose the therapeutical modality.

- **Saline sonohysterography** can identify and characterise the location of submucosal myomas missed on classical abdominal or transvaginal ultrasound.
- **Plain X-Rays of the lower abdomen and pelvis** usually identify only calcified fibroids and sometimes large fibroids may be seen as soft tissue or calcified masses displacing bowel gas [22].
- **Hysterosalpingography** may be useful in the infertile patient. It evaluates the contour of the uterine cavity and the patency of fallopian tubes but does not evaluate the exact location of fibroids.
- **CT scan** is not the investigation of choice, fibroids may be detected incidentally while investigating for another condition.

Laboratory investigations may reveal anaemia as a consequence of the menometrorrhagia of fibroids and depletion of iron stores or leucocytosis and raised C-reactive proteins in case of acute degeneration or infection.

Differential diagnoses of leiomyomas include pregnancy, adenomyosis, leiomyosarcoma, or solid ovarian neoplasms. Other conditions to be considered include sub involution, congenital anomalies, adherent adnexa, omentum or bowel benign hypertrophy, and sarcoma or carcinoma of the uterus [1]. The most common symptom of leiomyomata, recurrent abnormal bleeding, may be caused by any of the numerous conditions that affect the uterus. The definitive diagnosis in cases of uterine bleeding usually can be established by endometrial biopsy or fractional D&C [16].

6. Management

When uterine fibroids become symptomatic, medical or surgical treatment is offered to the patient, depending on her age, symptoms and future fertility desires.

A. Medical therapy includes:

- **Progestins**: Progestational therapy using norethindrone, medrogestone, and medroxyprogesterone acetate has been successful. These compounds produce a hypo-estrogenic effect by inhibiting gonadotropin secretion and suppressing ovarian function [17]. A small randomised controlled trial presented weak evidence of a reduction in fibroid size among women receiving lynestrenol compared with women receiving leuprolide acetate [13].
- **25 mg mifepristone** produces reduction in leiomyoma size and uterine volume and produces symptomatic improvement in women with fibroids [23].
- **Gonadotrophin Releasing Hormone (GnRH) agonists** have proven very useful for limiting growth or temporarily decreasing uterine fribroid's size. GnRH agonists induce hypogonadism through pituitary desensitisation, down-regulation of receptors, and inhibition of gonadotropins. They are however not suitable for long term use because they are associated with menopausal symptoms and bone loss but are likely to be beneficial preoperatively [24].
- **Oestrogen Receptors Modulators and Antagonists**: Because co-administration of oestrogen with progesterone was essential for growth and maintenance, inhibition of oesytogen receptors should also be an effective treatment for Leiomyomas [22].

B. Surgical therapies include:

- **Myomectomy:** There may be a beneficial effect of surgical resection of myomas to enhance fertility or successful pregnancy outcome [25]. It can be achieved using the following surgical procedures: open surgery, laparoscopy, robotic, transvaginal, and hysteroscopic surgery. The location and size of the myoma(s) dictates the specific surgical approach. Total abdominal myomectomy maintains fertility compared with hysterectomy but increases recovery time and postoperative pain compared with laparoscopic myomectomy [24]. However, there is high chance of recurrence with myomectomy, while hysterectomy is definitive. A rare complication of laparoscopic myomectomy is the occurrence of parasitic leiomyomas. They usually regress after menopause but in extremely rare cases they can calcify and present in a post-menopausal woman with atypical signs and symptoms [26].

- **Hysterectomy:** It is the procedure of choice whenever surgery is indicated for leiomyomas and when childbearing has been completed. It should also be considered in the event of a rapidly enlarging fibroids, in which a reasonable likelihood of malignancy exists. Different types of hysterectomies exist: laparoscopically-assisted vaginal hysterectomy, total vaginal hysterectomy, total abdominal hysterectomy and total laparoscopic hysterectomy. Total abdominal hysterectomy is considered to be beneficial in reducing fibroid-related symptoms, but total vaginal hysterectomy and total laparoscopic hysterectomy may have lower risks of complications, and shorter recovery times [18]. In 2010 Demir RH and Marchand GJ published a case report in which they resected a huge uterus weighing 3200 g via laparoscopic-assisted hysterectomy, laparotomy can be avoided in almost all instances of hysterectomy for benign disease for an experienced laparoscopic surgeon [27].

- **Uterine artery embolization (UAE):** It is the occlusion of the uterine artery, which reduces the blood supply to the uterus and ultimately to the uterine fibroids. There is evidence that uterine artery embolization patients are more likely to report greater improvements in symptoms, fewer complications and less additional interventions than myomectomy. Meanwhile, patients who undergo a myomectomy are more likely to have a conserved fertility [28, 29]. Complications of the technique include infections, complications of angiography and very rarely, uterine ischemia. However, there are no increased serious complications after UAE in patients with a large fibroid burden [30].

- **Laparoscopic occlusion of the uterine vessel**: It consists of cauterising the uterine artery at laparoscopy, with or without concurrent myomectomy. Based on the study of Helal et al. in 2010, both laparoscopic occlusions of the uterine vessel and embolization improve symptoms associated with uterine fibroids [31]. The laparoscopic procedure resulted in less postoperative pain and nausea and shorter hospital stays, although significantly more participants experienced heavy menstrual bleeding six months after laparoscopic occlusion, indicating a more favourable effect after uterine leiomyoma embolization. Thus, laparoscopic uterine artery occlusion is likely to attract considerable interest as an effective alternative to hysterectomy treatment of symptomatic uterine leiomyomata.

- **MRI- guided focused ultrasound surgery**. It was approved by the Food and Drug Administration (FDA) in October 2004 for the treatment of leiomyoma in premenopausal women who have completed childbearing. This outpatient procedure uses MRI for real-time thermal monitoring of the thermoablative technique, which concentrates multiple waves of ultrasound energy on a small volume of tissue to be destroyed [16]. Careful patient selection and use of pre-treatment imaging are important components for predicting the success of MR-guided focused ultrasound surgery of uterine leiomyomas [32]. Overall, there is reasonable tolerance, improvement in quality of life, and modest change in fibroid size. However, 11% of women experience worsened symptoms during more than a year of follow-up and 28% elect further treatment including myomectomy and hysterectomy [13].

7. Uterine Fibroids and Pregnancy.

The prevalence of leiomyomas in pregnancy varies between 10.7% to 16.7% [5, 33]. It's higher in African American women followed by Caucasians, Hispanic and Asian women [33]. According to a study done by Hasan et al. in 2010, fibroids are part of the factors predictive of bleeding in the first trimester of pregnancy and are also potential important predictors of heavy menstrual bleeding heaviness [34]. This is due to the oedema, increased vascularity and hypertrophy of uterine muscles that lead to the increase in size of fibroids during pregnancy. However, Laughlin et al. in 2010 think there could be a direct protective effect of pregnancy on fibroids after delivery. In their study of 171 postpartum women, they found that 36% of fibroids resolved to an undetectable level and those that remain were reduced in diameter by a median of 0.5 cm [35].

Generally, the effects of fibroids on pregnancy and labour are:

- Spontaneous abortion, especially with sub-mucousal leiomyomas due to the distortion of the uterine cavity and impairment of the vascular supply to the implanted ovum [36].

- Ectopic pregnancy if it interferes with the passage of the ovum.

- Incarceration of a retroverted gravid uterus in case of posterior wall uterine fibroid.

- Placenta praevia due to interference with implantation of the ovum in the upper uterine segment.

- Malpresentations; in the study of Tchente et al. in 2008, breech presentation was two times more encountered in pregnant women with fibroids [15].

- Abdominal discomfort if the tumour is large.

- Torsion of the uterus which is very rare and is found in subserousal fundal myoma.

- Premature or threatening premature delivery probably due to the stretching of the uterus by the fibroids or the liberation of prostaglandins and fever in red degeneration [15].

- Prolonged labour due to inertia from interference with normal uterine contractions.
- Obstructed labour in cervical myoma or pedunculated subserous myoma impacted in the pelvis.
- Postpartum haemorrhage due to interference with sub involution of the uterus and increased vascularity.
- Puerperal sepsis.

The management of uterine fibroids in pregnancy depends on the signs and symptoms:

In the majority of cases, no treatment is required. In case of pain, bed rest and narcotics are almost always successful [16]. Tocolytics may be necessary to control the uterine contractions in threatening premature labour. Myomectomy is generally contraindicated during pregnancy due to increased vascularity that may lead to haemorrhagic complications. However, laparoscopic myomectomy may be considered safe if done in early pregnancy but only in the hands of experienced laparoscopic surgeons [37]. Indications for it include red degeneration not responding to medical therapy, torsion of a pedunculated myoma or internal haemorrhage from rupture of a surface vein [36]. In case of obstructed labour, caesarean section is indicated but myomectomy is contraindicated. In the post-partum period, prophylactic antibodies should be given. Also, the women should be carefully observed for post-partum haemorrhage.

8. Conclusion

Uterine fibroids are the most frequent benign uterine tumours in females of reproductive age. Although benign in character they are associated with adverse outcomes such as miscarriages, aseptic necrobiosis, foetal mal-presentation, obstructed labour, premature births, caesarean sections, postpartum haemorrhage in pregnancy, and an altered menstrual cycle, heavy menstrual bleeding, infertility, constipation, urinary incontinence, and malignant transformation in non-pregnant women. Through this chapter the authors sought to contribute to the scarce evidence on its idiopathic pathophysiology and present all its available management options.

Author details

Joel Noutakdie Tochie[1,2]*, Gaelle Therese Badjang[3], Gregory Ayissi[3] and Julius Sama Dohbit[3]

1 Department of Anesthesiology and Critical Care Medicine, Faculty of Medicine and Biomedical Sciences, University of Yaoundé I, Yaoundé, Cameroon

2 Human Research Education and Networking, Yaoundé, Cameroon

3 Department of Obstetrics and Gynaecology, Faculty of Medicine and Biomedical Sciences, University of Yaoundé I, Yaoundé, Cameroon

*Address all correspondence to: joeltochie@gmail.com

References

[1] Pernoll ML. Benson and Pernoll's handbook of Obstetrics and Gynecology: Mc-Graw Hill Companies; 2001.

[2] Stewart EA. Uterine fibroids. Lancet. 2001;357(9252):293-8.

[3] Dohbit JS, Meka ENU, Tochie JN, Kamla I, Danwang C, Tianyi FL, Foumane P, Andze GO. Diagnostic ambiguity of aseptic necrobiosis of a uterine fibroid in a term pregnancy: a case report. BMC Pregnancy Childbirth. 2019 J;19(1):9.

[4] Lee CJ, Miller, E.S. DEJA REVIEW Obstetrics and Gynaecology: McGraw-Hill Companies; 2008.

[5] Egbe TO, Badjang TG, Tchounzou R, Egbe E-N, Ngowe MN. Uterine fibroids in pregnancy: prevalence, clinical presentation, associated factors and outcomes at the Limbe and Buea Regional Hospitals, Cameroon: a cross-sectional study. BMC Res Notes 2018;11:889.

[6] Huyck KL, Panhuysen CI, Cuenco KT, Zhang J, Goldhammer H, Jones ES, et al. The impact of race as a risk factor for symptom severity and age at diagnosis of uterine leiomyomata among affected sisters. Am J Obstet Gynecol. 2008;198(2):168 e1-9.

[7] Wise LA, Palmer JR, Stewart EA, Rosenberg L. Age-specific incidence rates for self-reported uterine leiomyomata in the Black Women's Health Study. Obstet Gynecol. 2005 ;105(3):563-8.

[8] Wise LA, Palmer JR, Spiegelman D, Harlow BL, Stewart EA, Adams-Campbell LL, et al. Influence of body size and body fat distribution on risk of uterine leiomyomata in U.S. black women. Epidemiology. 2005;16(3):346-54.

[9] Faerstein E, Chor D, Lopes Cde S. Reliability of the information about the history of diagnosis and treatment of hypertension. Differences in regard to sex, age, and educational level. The Pro-Saude study. Arq Bras Cardiol. 2001;76(4):301-4.

[10] Terry KL, De Vivo I, Hankinson SE, Missmer SA. Reproductive characteristics and risk of uterine leiomyomata. Fertil Steril. 2010;94(7):2703-7.

[11] Amanti L. S-BH, Abdollahi H., Ehdaeivand F. Uterine Leiomyoma and its association with menstrual pattern and history of progesterone acetate injections. International Journal of General Medicine. 2011;4:533-8.

[12] Ross RK, Pike MC, Vessey MP, Bull D, Yeates D, Casagrande JT. Risk factors for uterine fibroids: reduced risk associated with oral contraceptives. Br Med J (Clin Res Ed). 1986:9;293(6543):359-62.

[13] Viswanathan M, Hartmann K, McKoy N, Stuart G, Rankins N, Thieda P, et al. Management of uterine fibroids: an update of the evidence. Evid Rep Technol Assess (Full Rep). 2007;(154):1-122.

[14] Indranil CA, Shyamaoada D. Vaginal leiomyoma. Journal of Mid-Life Health. 2011;2(1):42-3.

[15] Tchente Nguefack C, Fogaing AD, Tejiokem MC, Nana Njotang P, Mbu R, Leke R. [Pregnancy outcome in a group of Cameroonian women with uterine fibroids]. J Gynecol Obstet Biol Reprod (Paris). 2009 ;38(6):493-9.

[16] DeCherney AHNL, Godwin TM, Laufer N, editor. Current diagnosis and treatments in Obstetrics and Gynaecology. Tenth ed: The Mc Graw-Hill Companies, Inc; 2007.

[17] Fortner KBSLM, Fox HE, Wallach EE, editor. The Johns Hopkins Manual of Gynaecology and Obstetrics. Third ed: Lippincott Williams and Wilkins; 2007.

[18] Hosseini H, Jacquemyn Y, Goossens K, Van Marck V. Atypical uterine leiomyoma: a rare variant of a common problem. BMJ Case Rep. 2009;2009.

[19] Okogbo FO, Ezechi OC, Loto OM, Ezeobi PM. Uterine Leiomyomata in South Western Nigeria: a clinical study of presentations and management outcome. Afr Health Sci. 2011;11(2):271-8.

[20] Hart R. Unexplained infertility, endometriosis, and fibroids. BMJ. 2003;327(7417):721-4.

[21] Dohbit JS, Meka E, Tochie JN, Kamla I, Mwadjie D, Foumane P. A case report of bicornis bicollis uterus with unilateral cervical atresia: an unusual aetiology of chronic debilitating pelvic pain in a Cameroonian teenager. BMC Womens Health 217;17(1):39.

[22] Wilde S, Scott-Barrett S. Radiological appearances of uterine fibroids. Indian J Radiol Imaging. 2009;19(3):222-31.

[23] Mukherjee S, Chakraborty S. A study evaluating the effect of mifepristone (RU-486) for the treatment of leiomyomata uteri. Niger Med J. 2011;52(3):150-2.

[24] Lethaby AE, Vollenhoven BJ. Fibroids (uterine myomatosis, leiomyomas). Clin Evid (Online). 2007;2007.

[25] Sinclair D, Gaither K, Mason TC. Fertility outcomes following myomectomy in an urban hospital setting. J Natl Med Assoc. 2005;97(10):1346-8.

[26] Hwang JH, Modi GV, Jeong Oh M, Lee NW, Hur JY, Lee KW, et al. An unusual presentation of a severely calcified parasitic leiomyoma in a postmenopausal woman. JSLS. 2010;14(2):299-302.

[27] Demir RH, Marchand GJ. Safe laparoscopic removal of a 3200 gram fibroid uterus. JSLS. 2010;14(4):600-2.

[28] Mara M, Maskova J, Fucikova Z, Kuzel D, Belsan T, Sosna O. Midterm clinical and first reproductive results of a randomized controlled trial comparing uterine fibroid embolization and myomectomy. Cardiovasc Intervent Radiol. 2008;31(1):73-85.

[29] Narayan A, Lee AS, Kuo GP, Powe N, Kim HS. Uterine artery embolization versus abdominal myomectomy: a long-term clinical outcome comparison. J Vasc Interv Radiol. 2010 ;21(7):1011-7.

[30] Smeets AJ, Nijenhuis RJ, Boekkooi PF, Vervest HA, van Rooij WJ, de Vries J, et al. Safety and effectiveness of uterine artery embolization in patients with pedunculated fibroids. J Vasc Interv Radiol. 2009;20(9):1172-5.

[31] Helal A, Mashaly Ael M, Amer T. Uterine artery occlusion for treatment of symptomatic uterine myomas. JSLS. 2010;14(3):386-90.

[32] Lenard ZM, McDannold NJ, Fennessy FM, Stewart EA, Jolesz FA, Hynynen K, et al. Uterine leiomyomas: MR imaging-guided focused ultrasound surgery--imaging predictors of success. Radiology. 2008;249(1):187-94.

[33] Laughlin SK, Baird DD, Savitz DA, Herring AH, Hartmann KE. Prevalence of uterine leiomyomas in the first trimester of pregnancy: an ultrasound-screening study. Obstet Gynecol. 2009;113(3):630-5.

[34] Hasan R, Baird DD, Herring AH, Olshan AF, Jonsson Funk ML, Hartmann KE. Patterns and predictors of vaginal bleeding in the first trimester of pregnancy. Ann Epidemiol. 2010;20(7):524-31.

[35] Laughlin SK, Schroeder JC, Baird DD. New directions in the epidemiology of uterine fibroids. Semin Reprod Med. 2010 ;28(3):204-17.

[36] El-Mowafi DM. Obstetrics Simplified. El-Happy Land Square, El-Mansoura, Egypt: Burg Abu-Samr; 1997.

[37] Ardovino M, Ardovino I, Castaldi MA, Monteverde A, Colacurci N, Cobellis L. Laparoscopic myomectomy of a subserous pedunculated fibroid at 14 weeks of pregnancy: a case report. J Med Case Rep. 2011;5(1):545.

Chapter 8

Herbal Medicine in Uterine Fibroid

Zi-Lin Li, Tung-Yung Huang, Yih Ho, Ya-Jung Shih, Yi-Ru Chen, Heng-Yuan Tang, Hung-Yun Lin, Jaqueline Whang-Peng and Kuan Wang

Abstract

Uterine fibroids, also known as uterine leiomyoma is the most common benign tumor of the uterus found in women of reproductive age. Uterine fibroids are the cause of major quality-of-life issues for approximately 25% of all women who suffer from clinically significant symptoms of uterine fibroid. Despite the prevalence of fibroid, currently, there are no effective treatment options for fibroid. The lack of understanding of the etiology of fibroid contributes to the scarcity of medical therapies available. Sex steroid hormones, dysregulation of cell signaling pathways, miRNA expression, and cytogenetic abnormalities may all implicate in fibroid etiology. Several herbal medicines have been used as anti-inflammation and antitumor agents. All of them have a common capability to inhibit expression of pro-inflammatory cytokines, proliferative genes, and pro-angiogenetic genes. Exploring herbal medicines as remedies lighten the hope of treatment. In the current review article, we discuss signal transduction pathways activated herbal medicines. We also address the possibility of using herbal medicines for uterine fibroid treatment.

Keywords: uterine fibroids, herbal medicines, curcumin, resveratrol, THSG, pycnogenol, AFE, EGCG

1. Background

Uterine fibroids are common benign muscle tumors of the uterus. It affects the normal life of thousands of women of childbearing age, especially non-Caucasian women, which can be caused by genetic and environmental factors. It is not usually fatal but can produce serious clinical symptoms. The prevalence of uterine fibroids is predicted to be approximately 70% depending on the population [1]. Clinical symptoms caused by uterine fibroid include pelvic pain or compression, abnormal uterine bleeding, gastrointestinal and voiding problems. It also produces pregnancy complications as well as fertility impairment. Since there are no effective medical therapies, invasive surgeries have become a clear option for the treatment of this tumor.

Studies on the whole genome of uterine fibroid indicate that there are many new signal transduction pathways and how gene nets play a role in uterine fibroid development. Not only in its origin, the transcriptomic, and epigenetic profiles, as well as the impact of the inter-cell matrix are all involved in uterine fibroid growth [2]. Additionally, microRNA plays a role in regulating uterine fibroid pathogenesis [3].

Nowadays, numerous treatments for fibroids are available. Therapies include conservative medications to invasive surgeries. Up to now, the regular therapy of uterine fibroid is surgery, but its negative impact on future fertility is evidenced. Therefore, selecting appropriate individualized therapy and augmented modifications to fit patient's expectations are readily important. However, newly developing pharmaceutical prospects have significant adverse effects, such as liver function impairment, hot flashes, bone density loss, endometrial changes, and inability to attempt conception during treatment [4].

Numbers of natural compounds are demonstrated effectively to treat uterine fibroids and to relieve their symptoms. In this review, we will discuss potential available herbal medicine compounds that may be beneficial for uterine fibroid patients, particularly those who plan to conceive during therapy or desire to preserve their future fertility. Nonetheless, there is still no significant clinic evidence available so far. Therefore, it is highly recommended to obtain more clinical trials utilizing these compounds before endorsing widespread usage [5].

2. Mechanisms and signal transductions in uterine fibroid

As the pathogenesis of uterine fibroids has not been fully elucidated, many studies have been carried out in mechanisms involved in this area and are still ongoing. The involved mechanisms affect several categories of cellular and tissue functions. The presumptive identification of progenitor stem cells of uterine fibroids has produced fibroids and maternal junctions, providing new clues about the etiology of uterine fibroids [2]. There are two hypotheses raised for the development mechanisms of uterine fibroid. However, they may cross-talk with each other intimately. The genetic hypothesis is focused primarily on the mutant mediator complex subunit 12 (MED12) genes [6], suggesting it onsets in the side population of the female reproductive system embryonic myoblasts and contributed rise to multiple small and medium fibroids later on [2]. Most studies on uterine fibroids have focused specifically on somatic mutations in the MED12 gene [6, 7]. According to the available data, this mutation has been confirmed in more than 70% of patients with uterine fibroids depending on different populations [6, 8]. Alternatively, the single and usually large-size fibroids are induced by predominantly epigenetic disorders in uterine fibroid steam cells, provoked by enhanced expression of the DNA hypomethylation in HMGA2 gene and epigenetic deregulation enhanced by hypoxia, muscle tension, or chromosome instability/aberrations (**Table 1**).

The life cycle of uterine fibroid is divided into two stages: transformation and benign tumor development [7, 57]. Mutations are sources for normal myometrial stem cells to transform into abnormal cells. Additionally, some other factors may also cause immunological changes [58] to lead to altered DNA repair and cell mutation [59]. Finally, a mixture of early environmental exposure and hyperreactivity to estrogen may also play a role in fibroid development [60].

Reactive oxygen species (ROS) formed after exposure to oxidative stress and/or hypoxia are linked to the activation of a variety of signal molecules [61–66]. Various enzyme systems produce ROS, including the mitochondrial electron transport chain, cytochrome P450, lipoxygenase, cyclooxygenase, NADPH oxidase complex, and peroxisomes [61]. Hypoxia triggers many key adaptive changes that enable cell survival, including inhibition of apoptosis, changes in glucose metabolism, and angiogenic phenotypes [61]. Recent studies have shown that oxygen depletion promotes mitochondria to increase more ROS production, and then activate signaling transduction pathways, such as hypoxia-inducible factor (HIF)-1α to promote cell survival and increase fibrotic growth sequentially [61].

	Curcumin	Resveratrol	THSG	Pycnogenol	*Anoectochilus formosanus*	EGCG
ERK1/2	Inhibition [9, 10] Activation [11]	Activation [12–15]	Inhibition [16] Activation	Decrease expression levels [17] Suppression [18]	Suppression [19]	Inhibition [20] Activation
PI3K	Inhibition [21]	Inhibition [22]	Inhibition [23, 24]	Activation [25]	NA	Activation [26] Inhibition [27]
NF-κB	Inhibition	Inhibition	Inhibition [16]	Suppression [18]	Activation [28] Inhibition [19, 29]	Inhibition [20, 30]
STAT3	Inhibition	Inhibition	NA	NA	NA	Inhibition [31]
AMPK	Activation	Activation	Activation [32]	Expression [33]	Activation [34, 35]	Activation [36, 37]
Nrf2	Activation	Activation	Activation [16, 32, 38]	NA	NA	Activation [39]
PPAR	Activation [40]	NA	Suppression [41]	Suppression [42]	Activation [36]	Activation
Suppression of gene expression	*PD-L, IL-1, IL-6, TNF-a*	*PD-L1, MMPs* [43]	*PD-L1*	NA	*PD-L1, COX-2, TNF-α, CAK, MMP-9,* and *TRAP* [29]	Proliferative genes [44]
Activation of gene expression	*Caspase-3, caspase-9*	*Caspase-3, caspase-9*	Apoptotic-related protein expression [24]	NA	Anti-proliferative genes [45, 46]	*BAX, p21, MDM2,* and *TP53I3* [30].
Anti-oxidant	Yes [47]	Yes	Yes [48]	Yes [33, 49]	Yes [19]	Yes [50]
Anti-inflammation	Yes	Yes	Yes	Yes [51]	Yes [45]	Yes
Anti-Cancer growth	Yes	Yes	Yes	Yes [52, 53]	Yes	Yes
ECM production inhibition	Yes [54]	Yes	Yes	NA	NA	Yes [55, 56]

THSG: 2,3,5,4'-Tetrahydroxystilbene-2-O-β-glucoside; EGCG: Epigallocatechin gallate; PPAR: Peroxisome proliferator-activated receptor; ECM: Extracellular matrix.

Table 1.
Signaling pathways, gene expressions and activities induced by natural products curcumin, resveratrol, THSG, pycnogenol, AFE and EGCG.

Remarkably, ovarian sex hormones play an important role in uterine fibroid pathophysiology [7, 67, 68]. Primarily under the influences of sex hormone, myometrial stem cells transform into pathological cells and develop into uterine lesions [69]. Tumor growth occurs by a large number of cell growth and extracellular matrix (ECM) building up [70, 71]. Accumulation and remodeling of ECM are believed to be crucial for fibrotic diseases such as uterine fibroid. Indeed, ECM plays an important role in forming the bulk structure of fibroids. Rigid ECM-rich structure may cause abnormal bleeding and pelvic pain [70, 72]. Therefore, a better understanding of ECM accumulation and remodeling is critical for developing new therapeutics for uterine fibroid. The ECM is approximate twice the volume in uterine fibroid compared to those in healthy myometrium. ECM is mainly composed of different types of collagen, fibronectin, and proteoglycan [70, 71]. It has been found in ultrafiltration that different fibers forming the ECM have abnormal structures and are different from the corresponding fibers in the unchanged tissue [73].

Estrogen has been shown to stimulate proliferation in a dose- and time-dependent manner in uterine fibroid cell lines [68, 74]. Estrogen (17β-estradiol) binds to the nuclear estrogen receptor (ER)-α to modulate the expression of proto-oncogenes, cytokines, and growth factors [75–77]. Uterine fibroid cells are more accessible to actions of 17β-estradiol than normal myometrial cells [78]. Although estrogen is essential for uterine fibroid growth, progesterone now is considered the key hormone to initiate uterine fibroid pathological differentiation and growth [7]. Estradiol has a tolerant effect on the growth of uterine fibroids mediated by progesterone. Additionally, the combination of estrogen and progesterone significantly increased cellular expression of the proliferation marker Ki-67 [79] and the accumulation of ECM due to the accelerated synthesis of type 1 and type 3 collagen [80]. Studies of Ishikawa et al. have shown that combined estrogen and progesterone increased uterine fibroid size more than 3-fold higher than those treated with estradiol alone or untreated controls in a xenograft model [67]. These results highlight the significant role of progesterone in uterine fibroid growth.

Furthermore, disturbance of steroid hormone receptors may be a primary pre-requisite for development of uterine fibroid [81]. Adenovirus-mediated a dominant-negative *ER*-α gene delivery eliminates the expression of estrogen and progesterone-regulated genes in uterine leiomyoma cells *in vitro* and shrinks uterine fibroids *in vivo* [82, 83]. Steroid hormones can affect uterine fibroid cells by different mechanisms including paracrine [7]. Steroid hormones stimulate expression of cytokines and growth factors. Sequentially, the induced cytokines and growth factors affect signal pathways, growth, and survival of uterine fibroid cells. They also regulate angiogenesis and ECM formation [84]. Consequently, this influences uterine fibroid cells to grow and survive and ECM to accumulate. ECM may serve as a reservoir for growth factors and cytokines to increase their stability and extend their influence [70].

Different growth factors and signal pathways are involved in uterine fibroid formation processes [71, 84]. As one of the most important growth factors affect development of uterine fibroid, transforming growth factor-β (TGF-β) stimulates uterine fibroid progress [71]. TGF-β signaling connects with other different pathways such as Smad pathway, phosphoinositide 3-kinase (PI3K)/Akt/mammalian target of rapamycin (mTOR), the mitogen-activated protein kinases (MAPK, ERK1/2) signaling cascade, and focal adhesion kinase (FAK) [71]. Expression of *TGF*-β is significantly increased in myometrial cells when they are directly in contact with the uterine fibroid tumor [85]. TGF-β1 stimulates expression of metalloproteinase-2 (*MMP-2*), *MMP-9*, and membrane-associated MMP inhibitor (*RECK*) [86]. TGF-β also modulates ECM production via cross-talk with growth factor and integrins [87, 88].

In addition to TGF-β, insulin-like growth factor–1 (IGF-1) is another growth factor that plays a vital role in the pathogenesis of uterine fibroid [89]. Studies of Boehm et al. indicated that more IGF-1 expression increases in uterine fibroid than in normal myometrium [90]. An animal model from Eker rat also showed upregulation of IGF-1 in uterine fibroid tissue [91]. We have shown how IGF-1R accumulated in uterine fibroid primary cell lines in response to IGF-1 to regulate cell proliferation [12]. Estrogen induces ERK1/2 activation and IGF-I, cell cycle regulating transcriptional factor A-Myb accumulation to stimulate uterine fibroid cell cycle progression in human uterine leiomyoma cell lines [92]. Additionally, growth hormone stimulates IGF-1 production to promote cell proliferation and to inhibit apoptosis in uterine fibroid [93, 94].

Wingless-type (Wnt)/β-catenin signaling also plays a role in somatic stem-cell function in both myometrium and uterine fibroid tissue [7]. Paracrine activation of the Wnt/β-catenin pathway in uterine fibroid stem cells can stimulate tumor growth [95]. Activin A, a product of macrophages, may also play a crucial role in uterine fibroid biology. Activin A is response for different immunological actions including cell transformation to lead to tumor development [58, 96]. Interactions between Wnt/β-catenin and TGF-β pathways, as well as with steroids and growth factors, give rise to the clonal formation of uterine fibroid tumors and are believed to be the basis of modern uterine fibroid biology hypothesis [7, 97].

The genetics of uterine fibroids and the etiology of epigenetic procedures have many peculiarities at first, then become quite similar and partially overlap due to the proximity of their genetic network and epigenetic environment. Research on the etiology of uterine fibroids to elucidate new strategies for the prevention and treatment of this common disease [2].

3. Treatment of uterine fibroid

Because the natural cause of uterine fibroid is not known, it makes the myomectomy or selected conditions hysterectomy to become the mainstay of management [98]. Genetic factors, epigenetic factors, and several pathogenic factors such as sex hormones, growth factors, cytokines, chemokines, and extracellular matrix components all of them have been implicated in development and growth of uterine fibroid [99, 100]. Although surgery has been suggested, it is not an attractive choice due to its serious consequences, especially with patients desiring to preserve their fertility potential [100].

Studies of El Andaloussi et al. [101] indicate that MED12 mutation presents a potential of dysregulating Wnt4/β-catenin to transform cells [101]. The dysregulating Wnt4/β-catenin affects mTOR signaling and caused autophagy abrogation, cell proliferation, and tumorigenesis [101]. Silenced MED12 gene reduces the proliferation of uterine fibroid cells [97]. In 2020, Ali et al. also found that β-catenin nuclear translocation contributes to uterine fibroid phenotype, and β-catenin signaling is modulated by estradiol and histone deacetylases activity [102]. Additionally, the Wnt/β-catenin pathway leads to increased levels of TGF-β3 [7, 71]. As we discussed above, different isoforms of TGF-β may play a crucial role in uterine fibroid development. Studies that used anti-uterine fibroid agents cause the attenuation of this pathway by reducing TGF-β3 signal and protein expression, resulting in a reduction in TGF-β canonical signaling [103]. Therefore, canonical Wnt pathway has been suggested to be a potential therapeutic target for the treatment of uterine fibroids [104].

It has been shown the proliferation of uterine fibroid is sensitive to the GnRH agonists [105, 106] or estrogen receptor antagonists. For those patients can be applied with hormone treatment with GnRH agonists including Lupron, Synarel, and Zoladex and/or aromatase inhibitors such as anastrozole (Arimidex®), letrozole (Femara®), exemestane (Aromasin®), vorozole (Rivizor®), formestane (Lentaron®), fadrozole (Afema®), and testolactone (Teslac®). Treatment with medications such as tamoxifen may also reduce uterine fibroid size [106]. In addition, using an adenovirus-expressing dominant-negative ER-α reduces ER-α to arrest fibroid growth in a mouse model which may provide an optional treatment [107]. Besides, alternative medicine has been shown to improve the symptom of uterine fibroids [108–110].

Alternatively, several natural products have been suggested for the treatment of uterine fibroids based on their natural activities of anti-inflammation, anti-proliferation, and anti-angiogenesis. We will discuss mechanisms in the following sections.

3.1 Curcumin

Curcumin is a yellow active natural polyphenol of the perennial herb *Curcuma longa,* commonly known as turmeric. In addition, curcumin is commonly found as ingredients in food seasoning, cosmetics, or herbal supplements. It has traditionally been used for decades in Asian countries as a medical herb due to its anti-microbial, anti-inflammatory, anti-tumorigenic, and anti-mutagenic properties [111]. Curcumin has many medical effects such as suppression of thrombosis [112], reduction of blood cholesterol [113, 114], and reduction of myocardial infarction [115]. Evidence indicates that curcumin suppresses the growth of several tumor cell lines [116, 117]. All in all, curcumin is effective against a variety of inflammatory illnesses and modulates multiple cell signaling pathways. However, it is still not well understood which binding site or receptor for it. *In vitro* studies indicate that curcumin can interact with integral components of cell signaling pathways and therefore may be pharmacologically relevant. However, only limited studies have shown functional consequences of curcumin interaction [118]. The tumor suppression mechanisms of curcumin are accredited by modulation of numerous targets playing important roles in tumor growth [119–122]. Those targets include transcription factors, receptors, kinases, cytokines, enzymes, and growth factors. Therefore, curcumin has been demonstrated to suppress the growth of several tumor cell lines [123]. It also inhibits the growth of uterine fibroid cells, even though there has yet to be a report describing the precise mechanism of its inhibition.

Curcumin inhibits phorbol ester-induced activation of NF-κB and ERK1/2 [9, 10]. Alternatively, it induces apoptosis via activation of ERK1/2 or SAPK/JNK in cancer cells [11]. Role of ERK1/2 activation in curcumin-treated cancer cells is controversial [124]. Curcumin down-regulates endothelial cell fibrosis and inhibits uterine fibroid cell proliferation via regulation of the apoptotic pathway, and it also reduced production of the ECM component fibronectin (**Figure 1**). Curcumin has also been shown to attenuate TGF-β-induced endothelial-to-mesenchymal transition [125]. Extracts from *Curcuma zedoaria* inhibits uterine fibroid cell proliferation compared to normal myometrial cells [126]. On the other hand, it stimulates caspase-3 and caspase-9 expression in uterine fibroid cells. Curcumin provides a novel direction for uterine fibroid therapies [127].

Peroxisome proliferator-activated receptor (PPAR) is a ligand-dependent transcription factor of the nuclear hormone receptor superfamily. It is expressed in a tissue-specific manner and plays an important role in the differentiation of adipocytes [128, 129]. PPARγ exerts anti-inflammatory, anticancer, and insulin sensitivity effects and participates in the control, proliferation, and differentiation

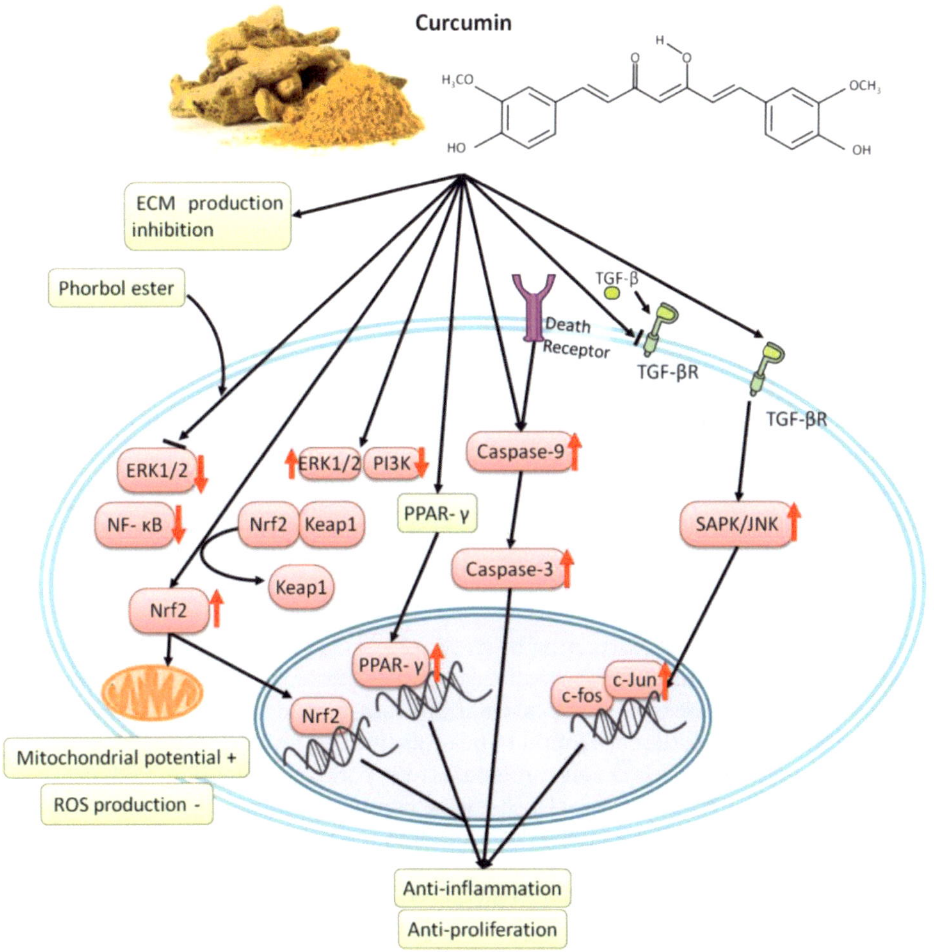

Figure 1.
Signaling pathways by which curcumin induces biological activities in cells. Curcumin binds to an unidentified cell surface binding site to activate the ERK1/2 cascade. On the other hand, in addition, to downregulate NF-κB activation, it inhibits phorbol ester-induced activation of NF-κB and ERK1/2. Curcumin also activates SAPK/JNK activation and Caspase-3 and -9-dependent apoptosis in cancer cells, may also including uterine fibroid cells. Curcumin inhibits TGF-β-induced ECM production. It also reduces inflammation and induces apoptosis.

of the cell cycle. Hepatic stellate cells are the type of hepatocyte responsible for fibrosis in liver damage and can lead to chronic liver damage and cirrhosis. Curcumin induces and activates PPARγ in rat hepatic stellate cells [40]. Curcumin considerably increases the proliferative inhibition of stellate cells by PPARγ. [40]. Besides, curcumin also enhances the activity of PPARγ in human colon cancer cell lines by reducing the expression of cyclin D1 and epidermal growth factor receptor (EGFR), thereby disrupting the cell cycle [130]. These two inhibitory effects depend on PPARγ activation. The study by Takashi Takeda et al. showed that uterine fibroids can share pathogenic characteristics with the development of metabolic syndrome [131]. PPARγ is also virtually involved in insulin signaling. A PPARγ agonist, thiazolidinedione, has been used to treat patients with type II diabetes [129]. Thiazolidinedione may be used to prevent the progression of atherosclerosis and metabolic syndrome [132]. On the other hand, curcumin directly inhibits fibroid proliferation, and curcumin-induced PPARγ activation can also prevent metabolic syndrome and indirectly inhibit fibroid growth [132]. However, since these findings were based on *in vitro* experiments, it raised concerns about the observation limitations. Later, Kenji Tsuiji et al. have developed a new *in vivo* uterine fibroid model to study the inhibition of rat leiomyoma (ELT-3) cells by curcumin [132]. The IC50 of curcumin-induced anti-proliferation in uterine fibroid cell lines is 20 μM, however, when patient-matched myometrial cells were exposed to equivalent concentrations of curcumin, there was no statistically significant inhibition of growth [127].

Studies indicated that curcumin absorption rate in the intestine is very low [133–136]. Similar raising concerns were also in other herb medicines, such as resveratrol discussed in next section. Thus, some modifications of curcumin need to be taken to keep its high blood concentration. Some studies regarding increased absorption and bioavailability of curcumin have been reported. For instance, the co-administration of curcumin and piperine can increase the bioavailability of curcumin [135]. Another strategy is to develop new curcumin analogues with a higher cell growth inhibitory capacity. One such compound, GO-Y030, has been shown to exhibit an 8- to 40-fold greater growth inhibitory potential than curcumin in several cancer cell lines [137, 138]. It may be useful to use the compound to clinically treat uterine fibroids.

3.2 Resveratrol

Polyphenols have been attracting by their anti-oxidative effects during the past years for human chronic diseases involved in inflammation like diabetes mellitus, neurodegenerative diseases, cardiovascular diseases, and cancers [139]. Resveratrol is one of well-studied stilbenes found in peanuts, grapes, and some berries. It is a plant product in response to environmental stress, pathogen infection, and ultraviolet radiation [127]. Resveratrol has been known as chemo-preventive, serving to suppress DMBA-induced ductal breast carcinoma [140] and ultraviolet light (UV)-induced skin cancer [141] in mouse models. Resveratrol induces p53-dependent apoptosis in several human cancer cell lines, including thyroid, prostate, and breast cancer cells [13, 142–145]. It also induces p53-independent anti-proliferation against cancer cells [14, 146–148]. Resveratrol has been recommended to be a reversion molecule for multiple drug-resistant breast cancer [149]. Resveratrol is safe and well-tolerated by patients, with common adverse events including nausea, diarrhea, and weight loss [150].

Although surface receptors involved in the resveratrol signal transduction remain to be identified, resveratrol binds to cell surface integrin αvβ3 to activate ERK1/2 and ant-proliferation in cancer cells [13, 145, 151] (**Figure 2**). Integrin αvβ3 is also involved in AKT phosphorylation [15, 152]. Resveratrol inhibits PI3K-AKT signal pathway to induce anti-proliferation [22] or other biological activities as IL-33-mediated mast cell activation [153].

Overexpression of integrin αvβ3 is observed in several types of solid tumors [154, 155] and highly growing endothelial cells [154, 155]. Our studies indicate that integrin αvβ3 overexpresses in primary uterine fibroid cell lines [12]. The integrin αvβ3 overexpresses in primary human uterine fibroid Case 016 and Case 018 compared to normal Case 003 cells [12]. Therefore, it is a perfect target for resveratrol which has been shown to bind on integrin αvβ3 receptor [13]. Integrins are not classic signaling receptors in that they possess no enzymatic activity. Integrin signaling depends on the allosteric behavior of the receptors, their ability to concentrate into adhesion zones, and the recruitment to these zones of numerous other adhesome components to form complex integrin-based cell adhesions [156, 157]. Many adhesome components are enzymes that interact with classic signaling pathways. Resveratrol regulates signal transduction via integrin αvβ3 in human uterine fibroid cells. Resveratrol attenuates expression of integrin αv and integrin β3

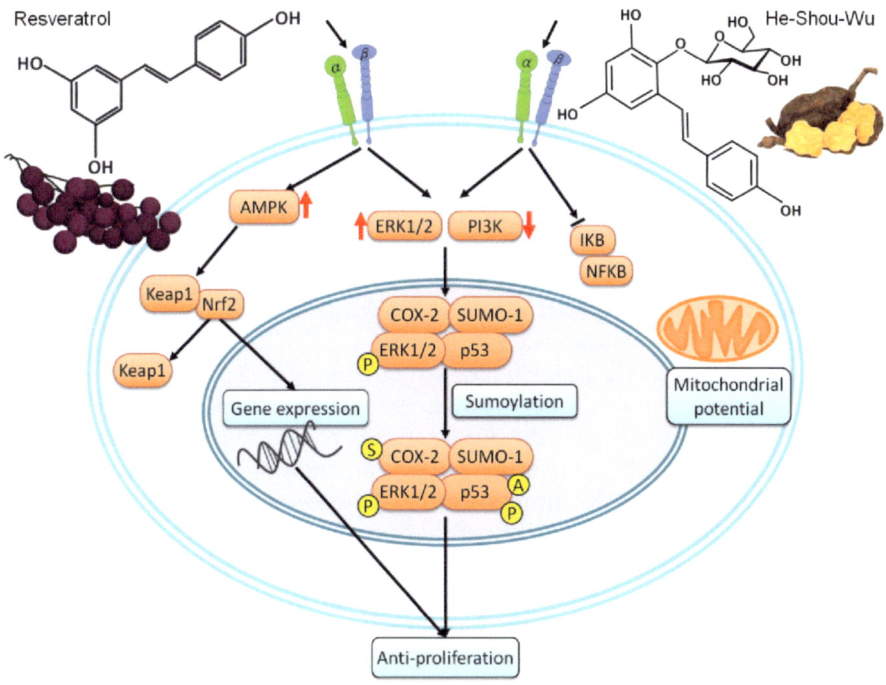

Figure 2.
Resveratrol/THSG activates signaling pathways in uterine fibroid cells. A stilbene receptor is present on integrin αvβ3 by which resveratrol activates ERK1/2 and induces nuclear accumulation of COX-2. On the other hand, 2,3,5,4′-tetrahydroxystilbene-2-O-β-glucoside (THSG) has a similar chemical structure and assumedly binds to integrin αvβ3 to activate the signal transduction pathway. In resveratrol-treated cancer cells, pERK1/2 also translocates to the cell nucleus and complexes with inducible COX-2. Phosphorylated ERK1/2 also translocates into the cell nucleus and forms a complex with inducible COX-2 in resveratrol-treated cancer cells. Resveratrol induces phosphorylation of the complexed p53 at Ser15 and p53-dependent antiproliferation. Blocking resveratrol-induced nuclear accumulation of COX-2 inhibits p53 phosphorylation and antiproliferation.

in primary uterine fibroid cell Case 016 and Case 018 but not in normal myometrial cells. Resveratrol induces ERK1/2 activation in uterine fibroid cells [12]. However, the constitutive phosphorylation of AKT in uterine fibroid cells was inhibited by resveratrol.

Integrin signaling and function are heavily dependent on cross-talk with other signaling pathways, especially growth factor signaling pathways [158–160]. Besides the aberrant integrin expression, IGF-1R highly expresses more in uterine fibroid compared to the normal tissues [161] indicating IGF-1 may also be involved in the abnormal proliferation [92, 162]. IGF-1 binds to IGF-1R to activate downstream AKT which is a target of resveratrol. Resveratrol did not inhibit IGF-1R phosphorylation in primary uterine fibroid cells [12]. These results suggest that the action of resveratrol on IGF-1R-dependent signal transduction is downstream IGF-1R at Akt level [12]. Resveratrol analogue, pterostilbene (3′,5′-dimethoxy-resveratrol) targets mTOR/PI3K/Akt signaling pathway to disrupt mitochondrial membrane potential, and induce apoptosis [163].

IGF-I mRNA is expressed significantly higher in leiomyoma cells than that in myometrial cells [12]. IGF-1 stimulates IGF-1R phosphorylation of but the action is blocked by resveratrol pre-treatment. Growth effect of IGF-1 can possibly reduce by resveratrol [164]. Resveratrol inhibits IGF-1-induced phosphorylated IGF-1R accumulation and proliferation consequently [12]. IGF-1 enhances leiomyoma cell proliferation and thereby accelerates uterine fibroid progression. In summary, resveratrol via a mechanism involved in crosstalk between integrin αvβ3 and IGF-1R-sensitive signal transduction pathways induces anti-proliferation in uterine fibroid.

Steroid hormones and thyroid hormone stimulate *TGF-β* expression [165]. Resveratrol blocks *TGF-β* expression and functions [166]. Cross talk among TGF-β signaling pathways, integrins, and ECM [88] is essential for uterine fibroid growth. Both Agarwal discussed the ability of resveratrol to infer with ECM formation and deposition in multiple diseases in their review article [53]. Resveratrol suppresses not only expression of fibronectin, fibromodulin, biglycan, and collagen types I and III, but also their protein levels in different cell lines [43]. Resveratrol also reduces MMP-9 protein accumulation but increases TIMP2 protein in ELT-3 cells and healthy uterine smooth muscle cells [43].

Resveratrol inhibits TGF-β signal downstream molecule AKT phosphorylation. Studies of confocal microscopy have shown resveratrol inhibits nuclear pAKT translocation in uterine fibroid cells. Alternatively, resveratrol does not interfere with pAKT nuclear translocation in normal uterine smooth muscle cells even though there are limited pAKT translocated [12]. Resveratrol reduces cellular levels of the phosphorylated/active form of anti-apoptotic kinase AKT in uterine cancer cells [167]. Sequentially, treatment of resveratrol reduces the endogenous cyclooxygenase-2 (COX-2) protein and produces PGE2 and PGF2α [167]. Evidence indicates that endogenous COX-2 is involved in inflammation, therefore, resveratrol inhibits AKT signaling pathway and COX-2 activity to induce anti-inflammation which plays vital roles in uterine fibroid cell growth.

β-catenin modulates and stimulates the stem cell renewal [168]. The regulation of the biologic functions for β-catenin is highly complex and not fully understood. Wnt proteins bind to a special cell-surface receptor, Frizzled, where it promotes activation of a cascade of proteins that leads to decreased β-catenin degradation in the cytosol and reduces nuclear β-catenin levels [7, 95]. The increased β-catenin expression is observed in uterine fibroids compared to the adjacent myometrium samples [169]. Ovarian steroids interact with the Wnt/β-catenin pathway to accelerate tumorigenesis [168]. Our studies also indicate that thyroid hormone increases nuclear β-catenin accumulation, thus β-catenin-dependent gene expression and proliferation [170, 171]. Resveratrol reduces expression and nuclear accumulation of β-catenin.

The expression of resveratrol-induced pro-apoptotic genes such as *COX-2* and *p21* induced in uterine fibroid cells. On the other hand, the expression of proliferative (anti-apoptotic) genes was either inhibited such as *BCL2*, and *CDKN2* or no changed as *Cyclin D1* and *PCNA*. The pro-apoptotic proteins such as caspase 3 and caspase 9, were also increased in resveratrol-treated cells [12]. Resveratrol-induced COX-2 facilitates p53-dependent anti-proliferation [172, 173]. Therefore, resveratrol induces anti-proliferation in uterine fibroid cells [12]. Kim et al. have also shown the extraction of herb medicine, *Scutellaria barbata D. Don* (*Lamiaceae*), down-regulates the IGF-I expression [174] and inhibits the proliferation of leiomyoma cells. *Scutellaria barbata D. Don* (*Lamiaceae*) induces the uterine smooth muscle cell differentiation markers in uterine smooth muscle cells and uterine leiomyoma smooth muscle cells, such as α smooth muscle actin (α-SMA), calreductin h1, and cyclin p27-dependent kinase inhibitor. In contrast, gene products linked to the G1 phase of the cell cycle, such as cyclin E and cdk2, are not affected by *Scutellaria barbata D. Don* (*Lamiaceae*) [175]. These observations agree with our studies. The expression of anti-apoptotic genes, such as *BCL2* and *CDKN2* are suppressed or unmodified *Cyclin D1* and *PCNA* [12].

Estrogen stimulates proliferation in breast cancer cells [176, 177], endometrial cancer [178, 179] and leiomyoma cells [180]. Estrogen also stimulates cell growth in uterine fibroid cells [12]. Resveratrol can inhibit estrogen-dependent cancer growth [176] and suppresses the proliferation of six sensitive uterine fibroid cases both in the absence and presence of estradiol [12]. These results indicate the suppressing effect of resveratrol on uterine fibroid growth may not go through ER-α.

The immunomodulatory factor, checkpoint PD-1/PD-L1 has been shown to play an important role in uterine fibroid pathogenesis. They also attack attention to be therapeutic targets. Resveratrol suppresses PD-L1 expression. In the presence of thyroid hormone, resveratrol traps PD-L1 in the cytosol, meanwhile, resveratrol-induced COX-2, an inducible transcriptional co-activator [181], is trapped with thyroid hormone-induced PD-L1 in the cytosol [173].

Summarily, in the primary cell culture of patients with resveratrol-sensitive primary uterine fibroids, resveratrol can inhibit uterine fibroid proliferation, induce apoptosis, and transmit integrin-dependent signaling αvβ3. The transduction pathway promotes uterine fibroids cell cycle arrest. Additionally, resveratrol inhibits the activation of IGF-1R dependent signal transduction pathways, which play an important role in uterine fibroid proliferation. Resveratrol may or may not inhibit the expression of proliferation genes. Resveratrol also induces the expression of p21 and COX-2. Analysis of the DNA content of the PI stain indicates that resveratrol induces uterine fibroid cells cell cycle arrest at sub-G1 population [12]. Crosstalk between αvβ3 integrin and IGF-1R plays a crucial role in resveratrol-induced uterine fibroid anti-growth. In addition, resveratrol inhibits signal transduction pathways and gene expression dependent on TGF-β and β-catenin. Therefore, resveratrol can effectively prevent leiomyoma overgrowth and treat uterine fibroids.

3.3 Extract of He-Shou-Wu, 2,3,5,4′-Tetrahydroxystilbene-2-O-β-glucoside

The stilbene glucoside 2,3,5,4′-tetrahydroxystilbene-2-O-β-D-glucoside (THSG) is one of the major bioactive components of *Polygonum multiflorum* Thunb (He Shou Wu). It is glycosylated resveratrol and it has been used as antiaging medicine [182]. THSG suppresses experimental colitis effectively by reducing the level of oxygen and nitrogen free radicals [48]. It also has been shown to exert a protective effect on cardiotoxicity induced by doxorubicin *in vitro* and *in vivo* [183]. THSG can also diminish peroxidation levels in the brain of a mouse model with Alzheimer's disease or cerebral ischemia–reperfusion. Administration of THSG not only prevents learning-memory deficits but also reverses the learning-memory deficit in disease-like mouse models with Alzheimer's [184].

Mechanism involved in *P. multiflorum*-induced anti-atherosclerosis may be caused by THSG-induced antagonistic effects on oxidation of lipoprotein, proliferation, and decrease of nitric oxide content of coronary arterial smooth muscle cells [185] which partially explains the antiatherosclerosis mechanism of *Polygonum multiflorum*. Recently, the pharmacological effects of *P. multiflorum* on atherosclerosis have been revealed with anti-inflammation and guy microbiota regulation of THSG in ApoE−/− mice [186]. The protective effects of THSG are mediated by modulation of JNK, SirT1, and NF-κB pathways [187] (**Figure 2**). As resveratrol, THSG can activate signal transduction pathways as AMPK. Treatment with THSG reduces the LPS-induced neuroinflammatory response, and that the mechanism by which THSG induces anti-neuroinflammatory effects may include the Nrf2/AMPK signaling pathways [38]. Consequently, THSG treatment leads to a decrease in the level of iNOS, TNF-α, and IL-6 production [184]. THSG-induced neuroprotective effects are via Akt signaling and TrkB activity [51]. THSG possessed an anti-inflammatory effect that may also be related to the inhibition of COX-2 enzyme activity and expression [188].

As a glycosylated analogue of resveratrol, THSG has similar effects as resveratrol. Studies indicate that resveratrol significantly stimulates cell proliferation of human gingival fibroblasts at low concentration (10 μM) but inhibited cell proliferation at high concentrations (100 and 200 μM) significantly. On the other hand, THSG significantly enhances growth of human gingival fibroblasts when the concentration is over 25 μM and does not show any cytotoxic effect in human gingival fibroblasts [151]. It is evidenced that THSG may not cause cytotoxicity in normal human cells. Although there are no studies regarding effect of THSG on uterine fibroid, it should be more effective than resveratrol. THSG may not enter cells to induce superoxide which causes cytotoxicity to cells. However, studies also indicate that crude extract may cause damage in hepatocellular cells.

3.4 Pycnogenol, French maritime pine bark extract

Pycnogenol is a standardized extract of the bark of French maritime pine. Pycnogenol is composed of flavonoids, mainly proanthocyanidins, and phenolic compounds. It is a known potent antioxidant [49]. Owing to the basic chemical structure of its components, the most obvious feature of pycnogenol is its strong antioxidant activity. In fact, phenolic acids, polyphenols, and in particular flavonoids, are composed of one or more aromatic rings bearing one or more hydroxyl groups. The compositions are hence potentially able to quench free radicals by forming resonance-stabilized phenoxyl radicals [189]. Pycnogenol is a strong antioxidant that may interfere with different pathways, and it plays an important role in diseases associated with oxidative stress. Hyperglycemia is characteristic of diabetic nephropathy and induces renal tubular cell apoptosis. Pycnogenol has been demonstrated to significantly suppress the high glucose-induced morphological changes and the reduction in cell viability associated with cytotoxicity in high glucose-treated renal tubular cells [49]. Pycnogenol is able to protect high glucose-induced apoptosis increasing Bcl2/Bax protein ratio level. Combination treatment of pycnogenol and metformin improves blood glucose levels, vascular reactivity, and left ventricular hypertrophy in induced diabetic rats [33]. Furthermore, combined treatment increases expression of AMPK, glucose transporter 4 (GLUT4), and calcium/calmodulin-dependent protein kinase II (CaMKII) in left ventricle of the hearts. However, the combination of these interventions has failed to possess higher efficacy [33].

Pycnogenol has anti-oxidative and anti-inflammatory efficacy in suppressing lipid peroxidation, total reactive species, superoxide $\cdot O_2$, nitric oxide NO·, peroxynitrite ($ONOO^-$), pro-inflammatory inducible nitric oxide synthase (iNOS) and COX-2 [49]. It also inhibits NF-κB nuclear translocation [49]. The safety of use of pycnogenol is demonstrated by the lack of side effects or changes in blood biochemistry and hematologic parameters. Therefore, pycnogenol has been recommended both for prevention and treatment of chronic venous insufficiency and related veno-capillary disturbances [190].

3.5 Therapeutic orchid *Anoectochilus formosanus* extract

Traditional herb medicine, golden thread (*Anoectochilus formosanus Hayata*) has been used to treat various diseases in Asia. *A. formosanus* extracts (AFEs) have been reported to possess hepatoprotective, anti-inflammatory, and anti-tumor activates. AFEs reduced blood glucose in hyperglycemic mice while there was no change in control group [191]. AFE and metformin at the same administrated dose of 50 mg/kg showed a similar effect on intraperitoneal glucose tolerance test in hyperglycemic mice. Free-radical scavenger capacity of AFE was concentration-dependent and 200 μg/ml of AFE was able to reduce more than 41% of the free radical [191]. The immunomodulatory protein from *A. formosanus* (IPAF) stimulated the TNF-α and IL-1β production, upregulated the expression of CD86, MHC II, IL-12, and

Th1-associated cytokines/chemokines [28]. It also enhanced the phagocytic activity of macrophages [28]. AFE inhibited constitutive *PD-L1* expression and its protein accumulation in cancer cells. AFE also induced expression of pro-apoptotic genes but inhibited proliferative and metastatic genes. Furthermore, it induced anti-proliferation in cancer cells. The results suggested that AFE not only reduced blood glucose concentration as metformin but also showed its potential use in cancer immune chemoprevention/therapy via hypoglycemic effect, ROS scavenging, and PD-L1 suppression [191]. In addition, IPAF stimulated expressions of TLR signal-related genes and the activation of NF-κB. IPAF could induce classically activated macrophage differentiation via TLR4-dependent NF-κB activation and had potential of IPAF to modulate the Th1 response [28].

3.6 Epigallocatechin gallate

The green tea polyphenol epigallocatechin gallate (EGCG) has not shown cytotoxicity to normal cells but induces apoptosis and growth inhibition of cancer cells [192, 193]. EGCG inhibits uterine leiomyoma cell growth *in vitro* and *in vivo*. The use of a green tea extract with 45% EGCG content has demonstrated clinical activity without side effects in women with uterine fibroid symptoms [194]. However, there are several shortcomings of EGCG including low stability, poor bioavailability, and high metabolic transformations under physiological conditions. All present challenges for its development as a therapeutic agent [194].

The signal transduction pathway by which EGCG exerts cell cycle arrest and induction of apoptosis remains to be clarified. Several mechanisms of cell-cycle arrest by EGCG have been postulated [195]. Transcription factor, p53 regulates downstream genes important in cell cycle arrest, DNA repair, and apoptosis. Loss of p53 in many cancers leads to genomic instability, impaired cell cycle regulation, and inhibition of apoptosis [196]. EGCG-treated HuLM cells exhibited increased expression of several genes that represent p53 pathway such as *BAX*, *p21*, *transformed 3 T3 cell double minute 2* (*MDM2*) and tumor protein p53 inducible protein 3 (*TP53I3*) [30]. The NF-κB signal pathway was impaired by EGCG and the expression of bcl2A1, a key factor in NF-κB pathway, was reduced 11.8-fold in 100 μM EGCG-treated uterine fibroid HuLM cells [30] compared to untreated control.

The BCL family includes proapoptotic members and antiapoptotic members, such as BAX and BCL-2, respectively. The effects of apoptosis or anti-apoptosis supplementary depend on the balance between BCL2 and BAX rather than on the BCL2 quantity alone [197]. EGCG treatment causes BCL2 to dramatically decrease while BAX up-regulates [30]. Additionally, the D-type cyclins, through the interaction with CDKs-forming cyclin d1-CDK4/6 complexes, are mainly responsible for driving the cell cycle from G1 to S phase [198]. A significant decrease was observed in the expression of CDK4 and PCNA in EGCG treated uterine fibroid HuLM cells [30].

4. Conclusion remarks

The current clinical uterine fibroid therapies are restricted to their short-term efficacy and unpleasant side effects. Unless the patients are postmenopausal, hysterectomy is generally not recommended. In terms of expanding medical options, alternative therapies for uterine fibroids have been explored. In addition to herbal medicines we discussed, natural products such as vitamin D, berberine, and others are being used for alternative uterine fibroid treatments. Moreover, it may be more effective when natural compounds combined with hormonal agents for uterine fibroid therapy. We have shown that resveratrol combined with thyroid hormone analogue, tetrac can compensate for resveratrol-induced RRM2 side effects in colorectal cancer animal xenograft model [199]. However, to search for a safe and effective medication for uterine fibroid requires further human clinical trials of these herbal compounds before promoting widespread usage.

Acknowledgements

The research described in this article from our team was supported in part by the Chair Professor Research Fund to Dr. K. Wang and Dr. J. Whang-Peng, by TMU Research Center of Cancer Translational Medicine from The Featured Areas Research Center Program within the framework of the Higher Education Sprout Project by the Ministry of Education (MOE) in Taiwan, by grants from the Ministry of Science and Technology, Taiwan (MOST107–2314-B-038-017 and MOST108–2314-B-038-050). We appreciate Miss Evelyn Yu-Chun Chen for her stunning proofreading expertise. The authors would like to extend their most sincere appreciation to Miss ABu and Miss Ya-Jung Shih for their prodigious research contributions from our group as mentioned in text.

Author details

Zi-Lin Li[1,2,†], Tung-Yung Huang[1,2,†], Yih Ho[3], Ya-Jung Shih[1,2], Yi-Ru Chen[1,2], Heng-Yuan Tang[4], Hung-Yun Lin[1,2,4,5*], Jaqueline Whang-Peng[1,6] and Kuan Wang[2]

1 Graduate Institute of Cancer Molecular Biology and Drug Discovery, College of Medical Science and Technology, Taipei Medical University, Taipei, Taiwan

2 Graduate Institute of Nanomedicine and Medical Engineering, College of Medical Engineering, Taipei Medical University, Taipei, Taiwan

3 School of Pharmacy, Taipei Medical University, Taipei, Taiwan

4 Pharmaceutical Research Institute, Albany College of Pharmacy and Health Sciences, Albany, NY, USA

5 TMU Research Center of Cancer Translational Medicine, Taipei Medical University, Taipei, Taiwan

6 Cancer Center, Wan-Fung Medical Center, Taipei Medical University, Taipei, Taiwan

*Address all correspondence to: linhy@tmu.edu.tw

† These authors contributed equally to this review article.

References

[1] Stewart, E. A.; Cookson, C. L.; Gandolfo, R. A.; Schulze-Rath, R., Epidemiology of uterine fibroids: a systematic review. BJOG **2017**, 124, (10), 1501-1512.

[2] Baranov, V. S.; Osinovskaya, N. S.; Yarmolinskaya, M. I., Pathogenomics of Uterine Fibroids Development. *Int J Mol Sci* **2019,** 20, (24).

[3] Jung, H. J.; Kim, H. J.; Park, K. K., Potential Roles of Long Noncoding RNAs as Therapeutic Targets in Renal Fibrosis. *Int J Mol Sci* **2020,** 21, (8).

[4] Sohn, G. S.; Cho, S.; Kim, Y. M.; Cho, C. H.; Kim, M. R.; Lee, S. R.; Working Group of Society of Uterine, L., Current medical treatment of uterine fibroids. *Obstet Gynecol Sci* **2018,** 61, (2), 192-201.

[5] Ciebiera, M.; Ali, M.; Prince, L.; Jackson-Bey, T.; Atabiekov, I.; Zgliczynski, S.; Al-Hendy, A., The Evolving Role of Natural Compounds in the Medical Treatment of Uterine Fibroids. *J Clin Med* **2020,** 9, (5).

[6] Makinen, N.; Mehine, M.; Tolvanen, J.; Kaasinen, E.; Li, Y.; Lehtonen, H. J.; Gentile, M.; Yan, J.; Enge, M.; Taipale, M.; Aavikko, M.; Katainen, R.; Virolainen, E.; Bohling, T.; Koski, T. A.; Launonen, V.; Sjoberg, J.; Taipale, J.; Vahteristo, P.; Aaltonen, L. A., MED12, the mediator complex subunit 12 gene, is mutated at high frequency in uterine leiomyomas. *Science* **2011,** 334, (6053), 252-5.

[7] Bulun, S. E., Uterine fibroids. *N Engl J Med* **2013,** 369, (14), 1344-55.

[8] Halder, S. K.; Laknaur, A.; Miller, J.; Layman, L. C.; Diamond, M.; Al-Hendy, A., Novel MED12 gene somatic mutations in women from the Southern United States with symptomatic uterine fibroids. *Mol Genet Genomics* **2015,** 290, (2), 505-11.

[9] Chun, K. S.; Keum, Y. S.; Han, S. S.; Song, Y. S.; Kim, S. H.; Surh, Y. J., Curcumin inhibits phorbol ester-induced expression of cyclooxygenase-2 in mouse skin through suppression of extracellular signal-regulated kinase activity and NF-kappaB activation. *Carcinogenesis* **2003,** 24, (9), 1515-24.

[10] Olivera, A.; Moore, T. W.; Hu, F.; Brown, A. P.; Sun, A.; Liotta, D. C.; Snyder, J. P.; Yoon, Y.; Shim, H.; Marcus, A. I.; Miller, A. H.; Pace, T. W., Inhibition of the NF-kappaB signaling pathway by the curcumin analog, 3,5-Bis(2-pyridinylmethylidene)-4-piperidone (EF31): anti-inflammatory and anti-cancer properties. *Int Immunopharmacol* **2012,** 12, (2), 368-77.

[11] Lim, W.; Jeong, M.; Bazer, F. W.; Song, G., Curcumin Suppresses Proliferation and Migration and Induces Apoptosis on Human Placental Choriocarcinoma Cells via ERK1/2 and SAPK/JNK MAPK Signaling Pathways. *Biol Reprod* **2016,** 95, (4), 83.

[12] Ho, Y.; Sh Yang, Y. C.; Chin, Y. T.; Chou, S. Y.; Chen, Y. R.; Shih, Y. J.; Whang-Peng, J.; Changou, C. A.; Liu, H. L.; Lin, S. J.; Tang, H. Y.; Lin, H. Y.; Davis, P. J., Resveratrol inhibits human leiomyoma cell proliferation via crosstalk between integrin alphavbeta3 and IGF-1R. *Food Chem Toxicol* **2018,** 120, 346-355.

[13] Chin, Y. T.; Hsieh, M. T.; Yang, S. H.; Tsai, P. W.; Wang, S. H.; Wang, C. C.; Lee, Y. S.; Cheng, G. Y.; HuangFu, W. C.; London, D.; Tang, H. Y.; Fu, E.; Yen, Y.; Liu, L. F.; Lin, H. Y.; Davis, P. J., Anti-proliferative and gene expression actions of resveratrol in breast cancer cells in vitro. *Oncotarget* **2014,** 5, (24), 12891-907.

[14] Gosslau, A.; Pabbaraja, S.; Knapp, S.; Chen, K. Y., Trans- and cis-stilbene polyphenols induced rapid perinuclear mitochondrial clustering and p53-independent apoptosis in cancer cells but not normal cells. *Eur J Pharmacol* **2008,** 587, (1-3), 25-34.

[15] Hwang, S.; Lee, H. J.; Kim, G.; Won, K. J.; Park, Y. S.; Jo, I., CCN1 acutely increases nitric oxide production via integrin alphavbeta3-Akt-S6K-phosphorylation of endothelial nitric oxide synthase at the serine 1177 signaling axis. *Free Radic Biol Med* **2015,** 89, 229-40.

[16] Park, S. Y.; Jin, M. L.; Kang, N. J.; Park, G.; Choi, Y. W., Anti-inflammatory effects of novel *Polygonum multiflorum* compound via inhibiting NF-kappaB/MAPK and upregulating the Nrf2 pathways in LPS-stimulated microglia. *Neurosci Lett* **2017,** 651, 43-51.

[17] Shin, N. R.; Ryu, H. W.; Ko, J. W.; Park, J. W.; Kwon, O. K.; Oh, S. R.; Kim, J. C.; Shin, I. S.; Ahn, K. S., A standardized bark extract of *Pinus pinaster* Aiton (Pycnogenol((R))) attenuated chronic obstructive pulmonary disease via Erk-sp1 signaling pathway. *J Ethnopharmacol* **2016,** 194, 412-420.

[18] Xia, R.; Ji, C.; Zhang, L., Neuroprotective Effects of Pycnogenol Against Oxygen-Glucose Deprivation/Reoxygenation-Induced Injury in Primary Rat Astrocytes via NF-kappaB and ERK1/2 MAPK Pathways. *Cell Physiol Biochem* **2017,** 42, (3), 987-998.

[19] Hsieh, W. T.; Tsai, C. T.; Wu, J. B.; Hsiao, H. B.; Yang, L. C.; Lin, W. C., Kinsenoside, a high yielding constituent from Anoectochilus formosanus, inhibits carbon tetrachloride induced Kupffer cells mediated liver damage. *J Ethnopharmacol* **2011,** 135, (2), 440-9.

[20] Liang, Y.; Ip, M. S. M.; Mak, J. C. W., (-)-Epigallocatechin-3-gallate suppresses cigarette smoke-induced inflammation in human cardiomyocytes via ROS-mediated MAPK and NF-kappaB pathways. *Phytomedicine* **2019,** 58, 152768.

[21] Hamzehzadeh, L.; Atkin, S. L.; Majeed, M.; Butler, A. E.; Sahebkar, A., The versatile role of curcumin in cancer prevention and treatment: A focus on PI3K/AKT pathway. *J Cell Physiol* **2018,** 233, (10), 6530-6537.

[22] Chai, R.; Fu, H.; Zheng, Z.; Liu, T.; Ji, S.; Li, G., Resveratrol inhibits proliferation and migration through SIRT1 mediated posttranslational modification of PI3K/AKT signaling in hepatocellular carcinoma cells. *Mol Med Rep* **2017,** 16, (6), 8037-8044.

[23] Yang, X. P.; Liu, T. Y.; Qin, X. Y.; Yu, L. C., Potential protection of 2,3,5,4′-tetrahydroxystilbene-2-O-beta-D-glucoside against staurosporine-induced toxicity on cultured rat hippocampus neurons. *Neurosci Lett* **2014,** 576, 79-83.

[24] Shen, J.; Zhang, Y.; Shen, H.; Pan, H.; Xu, L.; Yuan, L.; Ding, Z., The synergistic effect of 2,3,5,4'-Tetrahydroxystilbene-2-O-beta-d-glucoside combined with Adriamycin on MCF-7 breast cancer cells. *Drug Des Devel Ther* **2018,** 12, 4083-4094.

[25] Lee, H. H.; Kim, K. J.; Lee, O. H.; Lee, B. Y., Effect of pycnogenol on glucose transport in mature 3T3-L1 adipocytes. *Phytother Res* **2010,** 24, (8), 1242-9.

[26] Jamuna, S.; Ashokkumar, R.; Sakeena Sadullah, M. S.; Devaraj, S. N., Oligomeric proanthocyanidins and epigallocatechin gallate aggravate autophagy of foam cells through the activation of Class III PI3K/Beclin1-complex mediated cholesterol efflux. *Biofactors* **2019,** 45, (5), 763-773.

[27] Gu, J. J.; Qiao, K. S.; Sun, P.; Chen, P.; Li, Q., Study of EGCG induced

apoptosis in lung cancer cells by inhibiting PI3K/Akt signaling pathway. *Eur Rev Med Pharmacol Sci* **2018,** 22, (14), 4557-4563.

[28] Kuan, Y. C.; Lee, W. T.; Hung, C. L.; Yang, C.; Sheu, F., Investigating the function of a novel protein from Anoectochilus formosanus which induced macrophage differentiation through TLR4-mediated NF-kappaB activation. *Int Immunopharmacol* **2012,** 14, (1), 114-20.

[29] Hsiao, H. B.; Lin, H.; Wu, J. B.; Lin, W. C., Kinsenoside prevents ovariectomy-induced bone loss and suppresses osteoclastogenesis by regulating classical NF-kappaB pathways. *Osteoporos Int* **2013,** 24, (5), 1663-76.

[30] Zhang, D.; Al-Hendy, M.; Richard-Davis, G.; Montgomery-Rice, V.; Rajaratnam, V.; Al-Hendy, A., Antiproliferative and proapoptotic effects of epigallocatechin gallate on human leiomyoma cells. *Fertil Steril* **2010,** 94, (5), 1887-93.

[31] Wang, Y.; Ren, X.; Deng, C.; Yang, L.; Yan, E.; Guo, T.; Li, Y.; Xu, M. X., Mechanism of the inhibition of the STAT3 signaling pathway by EGCG. *Oncol Rep* **2013,** 30, (6), 2691-6.

[32] Park, S. Y.; Jin, M. L.; Chae, S. Y.; Ko, M. J.; Choi, Y. H.; Park, G.; Choi, Y. W., Novel compound from *Polygonum multiflorum* inhibits inflammatory response in LPS-stimulated microglia by upregulating AMPK/Nrf2 pathways. *Neurochem Int* **2016,** 100, 21-29.

[33] Jankyova, S.; Rubintova, D.; Janosikova, L.; Panek, P.; Foltanova, T.; Kralova, E., The Effects of Pycnogenol(R) as Add-on Drug to Metformin Therapy in Diabetic Rats. *Phytother Res* **2016,** 30, (8), 1354-61.

[34] Lee, Y. G.; Sue, Y. M.; Lee, C. K.; Huang, H. M.; He, J. J.; Wang, Y. S.; Juan, S. H., Synergistic effects of cAMP-dependent protein kinase A and AMP-activated protein kinase on lipolysis in kinsenoside-treated C3H10T1/2 adipocytes. *Phytomedicine* **2019,** 55, 255-263.

[35] Cheng, K. T.; Wang, Y. S.; Chou, H. C.; Chang, C. C.; Lee, C. K.; Juan, S. H., Kinsenoside-mediated lipolysis through an AMPK-dependent pathway in C3H10T1/2 adipocytes: Roles of AMPK and PPARalpha in the lipolytic effect of kinsenoside. *Phytomedicine* **2015,** 22, (6), 641-7.

[36] Li, B.; Takeda, T.; Tsuiji, K.; Kondo, A.; Kitamura, M.; Wong, T. F.; Yaegashi, N., The antidiabetic drug metformin inhibits uterine leiomyoma cell proliferation via an AMP-activated protein kinase signaling pathway. *Gynecol Endocrinol* **2013,** 29, (1), 87-90.

[37] Ueda-Wakagi, M.; Hayashibara, K.; Nagano, T.; Ikeda, M.; Yuan, S.; Ueda, S.; Shirai, Y.; Yoshida, K. I.; Ashida, H., Epigallocatechin gallate induces GLUT4 translocation in skeletal muscle through both PI3K- and AMPK-dependent pathways. *Food Funct* **2018,** 9, (8), 4223-4233.

[38] Park, S. Y.; Jin, M. L.; Wang, Z.; Park, G.; Choi, Y. W., 2,3,4′,5-tetrahydroxystilbene-2-O-beta-d-glucoside exerts anti-inflammatory effects on lipopolysaccharide-stimulated microglia by inhibiting NF-kappaB and activating AMPK/Nrf2 pathways. *Food Chem Toxicol* **2016,** 97, 159-167.

[39] Pan, C.; Zhou, S.; Wu, J.; Liu, L.; Song, Y.; Li, T.; Ha, L.; Liu, X.; Wang, F.; Tian, J.; Wu, H., NRF2 Plays a Critical Role in Both Self and EGCG Protection against Diabetic Testicular Damage. *Oxid Med Cell Longev* **2017,** 2017, 3172692.

[40] Xu, J.; Fu, Y.; Chen, A., Activation of peroxisome proliferator-activated receptor-gamma contributes to the

inhibitory effects of curcumin on rat hepatic stellate cell growth. *Am J Physiol Gastrointest Liver Physiol* **2003,** 285, (1), G20-30.

[41] Meng, Y. K.; Li, C. Y.; Li, R. Y.; He, L. Z.; Cui, H. R.; Yin, P.; Zhang, C. E.; Li, P. Y.; Sang, X. X.; Wang, Y.; Niu, M.; Zhang, Y. M.; Guo, Y. M.; Sun, R.; Wang, J. B.; Bai, Z. F.; Xiao, X. H., Cis-stilbene glucoside in *Polygonum multiflorum* induces immunological idiosyncratic hepatotoxicity in LPS-treated rats by suppressing PPAR-gamma. *Acta Pharmacol Sin* **2017,** 38, (10), 1340-1352.

[42] Lee, O. H.; Seo, M. J.; Choi, H. S.; Lee, B. Y., Pycnogenol(R) inhibits lipid accumulation in 3T3-L1 adipocytes with the modulation of reactive oxygen species (ROS) production associated with antioxidant enzyme responses. *Phytother Res* **2012,** 26, (3), 403-11.

[43] Wu, C. H.; Shieh, T. M.; Wei, L. H.; Cheng, T. F.; Chen, H. Y.; Huang, T. C.; Wang, K. L.; Hsai, S. M., Resveratrol inhibits proliferation of myometrial and leiomyoma cells and decreases extracellular matrix-associated protein expression. *Journal of Functional Foods* **2016,** 23, 12.

[44] Wang, S. I.; Mukhtar, H., Gene expression profile in human prostate LNCaP cancer cells by (--) epigallocatechin-3-gallate. *Cancer Lett* **2002,** 182, (1), 43-51.

[45] Yang, L. C.; Hsieh, C. C.; Lu, T. J.; Lin, W. C., Structurally characterized arabinogalactan from Anoectochilus formosanus as an immuno-modulator against CT26 colon cancer in BALB/c mice. *Phytomedicine* **2014,** 21, (5), 647-55.

[46] Shyur, L. F.; Chen, C. H.; Lo, C. P.; Wang, S. Y.; Kang, P. L.; Sun, S. J.; Chang, C. A.; Tzeng, C. M.; Yang, N. S., Induction of apoptosis in MCF-7 human breast cancer cells by phytochemicals from Anoectochilus formosanus. *J Biomed Sci* **2004,** 11, (6), 928-39.

[47] Arshad, L.; Haque, M. A.; Abbas Bukhari, S. N.; Jantan, I., An overview of structure-activity relationship studies of curcumin analogs as antioxidant and anti-inflammatory agents. *Future Med Chem* **2017,** 9, (6), 605-626.

[48] Wang, X.; Zhao, L.; Han, T.; Chen, S.; Wang, J., Protective effects of 2,3,5,4′-tetrahydroxystilbene-2-O-beta-d-glucoside, an active component of *Polygonum multiflorum* Thunb, on experimental colitis in mice. *Eur J Pharmacol* **2008,** 578, (2-3), 339-48.

[49] Kim, Y. J.; Kim, Y. A.; Yokozawa, T., Pycnogenol modulates apoptosis by suppressing oxidative stress and inflammation in high glucose-treated renal tubular cells. *Food Chem Toxicol* **2011,** 49, (9), 2196-201.

[50] Pan, H.; Chen, J.; Shen, K.; Wang, X.; Wang, P.; Fu, G.; Meng, H.; Wang, Y.; Jin, B., Mitochondrial modulation by Epigallocatechin 3-Gallate ameliorates cisplatin induced renal injury through decreasing oxidative/nitrative stress, inflammation and NF-kB in mice. *PLoS One* **2015,** 10, (4), e0124775.

[51] Yu, Y.; Lang, X. Y.; Li, X. X.; Gu, R. Z.; Liu, Q. S.; Lan, R.; Qin, X. Y., 2,3,5,4'-Tetrahydroxystilbene-2-O-beta-d-glucoside attenuates MPP+/MPTP-induced neurotoxicity in vitro and in vivo by restoring the BDNF-TrkB and FGF2-Akt signaling axis and inhibition of apoptosis. *Food Funct* **2019,** 10, (9), 6009-6019.

[52] Huang, W. W.; Yang, J. S.; Lin, C. F.; Ho, W. J.; Lee, M. R., Pycnogenol induces differentiation and apoptosis in human promyeloid leukemia HL-60 cells. *Leuk Res* **2005,** 29, (6), 685-92.

[53] Harati, K.; Slodnik, P.; Chromik, A. M.; Behr, B.; Goertz, O.; Hirsch, T.; Kapalschinski, N.; Klein-Hitpass, L.;

Kolbenschlag, J.; Uhl, W.; Lehnhardt, M.; Daigeler, A., Proapoptotic effects of pycnogenol on HT1080 human fibrosarcoma cells. *Int J Oncol* **2015,** 46, (4), 1629-36.

[54] Agarwal, R.; Agarwal, P., Targeting extracellular matrix remodeling in disease: Could resveratrol be a potential candidate? *Exp Biol Med (Maywood)* **2017,** 242, (4), 374-383.

[55] Lee, J. H.; Chung, J. H.; Cho, K. H., The effects of epigallocatechin-3-gallate on extracellular matrix metabolism. *J Dermatol Sci* **2005,** 40, (3), 195-204.

[56] Han, Y.; Wang, Q.; Fan, X.; Chu, J.; Peng, J.; Zhu, Y.; Li, Y.; Li, X.; Shen, L.; Asenso, J.; Li, S., Epigallocatechin gallate attenuates overloadinduced cardiac ECM remodeling via restoring T cell homeostasis. *Mol Med Rep* **2017,** 16, (3), 3542-3550.

[57] McWilliams, M. M.; Chennathukuzhi, V. M., Recent Advances in Uterine Fibroid Etiology. *Semin Reprod Med* **2017,** 35, (2), 181-189.

[58] Protic, O.; Toti, P.; Islam, M. S.; Occhini, R.; Giannubilo, S. R.; Catherino, W. H.; Cinti, S.; Petraglia, F.; Ciavattini, A.; Castellucci, M.; Hinz, B.; Ciarmela, P., Possible involvement of inflammatory/reparative processes in the development of uterine fibroids. *Cell Tissue Res* **2016,** 364, (2), 415-27.

[59] Elhusseini, H.; Elkafas, H.; Abdelaziz, M.; Halder, S.; Atabiekov, I.; Eziba, N.; Ismail, N.; El Andaloussi, A.; Al-Hendy, A., Diet-induced vitamin D deficiency triggers inflammation and DNA damage profile in murine myometrium. *Int J Womens Health* **2018,** 10, 503-514.

[60] Yang, Q.; Diamond, M. P.; Al-Hendy, A., Early Life Adverse Environmental Exposures Increase the Risk of Uterine Fibroid Development: Role of Epigenetic Regulation. *Front Pharmacol* **2016,** 7, 40.

[61] Fruehauf, J. P.; Meyskens, F. L., Jr., Reactive oxygen species: a breath of life or death? *Clin Cancer Res* **2007,** 13, (3), 789-94.

[62] Halliwell, B., Reactive oxygen species in living systems: source, biochemistry, and role in human disease. *Am J Med* **1991,** 91, (3C), 14S–22S.

[63] Harris, A. L., Hypoxia--a key regulatory factor in tumour growth. *Nat Rev Cancer* **2002,** 2, (1), 38-47.

[64] Inoue, M.; Sato, E. F.; Nishikawa, M.; Park, A. M.; Kira, Y.; Imada, I.; Utsumi, K., Mitochondrial generation of reactive oxygen species and its role in aerobic life. *Curr Med Chem* **2003,** 10, (23), 2495-505.

[65] Kamata, H.; Hirata, H., Redox regulation of cellular signalling. *Cell Signal* **1999,** 11, (1), 1-14.

[66] Kieran, M. W.; Folkman, J.; Heymach, J., Angiogenesis inhibitors and hypoxia. *Nat Med* **2003,** 9, (9), 1104; author reply 1104-5.

[67] Ishikawa, H.; Ishi, K.; Serna, V. A.; Kakazu, R.; Bulun, S. E.; Kurita, T., Progesterone is essential for maintenance and growth of uterine leiomyoma. *Endocrinology* **2010,** 151, (6), 2433-42.

[68] Borahay, M. A.; Al-Hendy, A.; Kilic, G. S.; Boehning, D., Signaling Pathways in Leiomyoma: Understanding Pathobiology and Implications for Therapy. *Mol Med* **2015,** 21, 242-56.

[69] Ono, M.; Qiang, W.; Serna, V. A.; Yin, P.; Coon, J. S. t.; Navarro, A.; Monsivais, D.; Kakinuma, T.; Dyson, M.; Druschitz, S.; Unno, K.; Kurita, T.; Bulun, S. E., Role of stem cells in human

uterine leiomyoma growth. *PLoS One* **2012,** 7, (5), e36935.

[70] Islam, M. S.; Ciavattini, A.; Petraglia, F.; Castellucci, M.; Ciarmela, P., Extracellular matrix in uterine leiomyoma pathogenesis: a potential target for future therapeutics. *Hum Reprod Update* **2018,** 24, (1), 59-85.

[71] Kudo, D.; Suto, A.; Hakamada, K., The Development of a Novel Therapeutic Strategy to Target Hyaluronan in the Extracellular Matrix of Pancreatic Ductal Adenocarcinoma. *Int J Mol Sci* **2017,** 18, (3).

[72] Islam, M. S.; Akhtar, M. M.; Segars, J. H.; Castellucci, M.; Ciarmela, P., Molecular targets of dietary phytochemicals for possible prevention and therapy of uterine fibroids: Focus on fibrosis. *Crit Rev Food Sci Nutr* **2017,** 57, (17), 3583-3600.

[73] Sozen, I.; Arici, A., Interactions of cytokines, growth factors, and the extracellular matrix in the cellular biology of uterine leiomyomata. *Fertil Steril* **2002,** 78, (1), 1-12.

[74] Al-Hendy, A.; Diamond, M. P.; El-Sohemy, A.; Halder, S. K., 1,25-dihydroxyvitamin D3 regulates expression of sex steroid receptors in human uterine fibroid cells. *J Clin Endocrinol Metab* **2015,** 100, (4), E572-82.

[75] Curtis, S. W.; Washburn, T.; Sewall, C.; DiAugustine, R.; Lindzey, J.; Couse, J. F.; Korach, K. S., Physiological coupling of growth factor and steroid receptor signaling pathways: estrogen receptor knockout mice lack estrogen-like response to epidermal growth factor. *Proc Natl Acad Sci U S A* **1996,** 93, (22), 12626-30.

[76] Nilsson, S.; Makela, S.; Treuter, E.; Tujague, M.; Thomsen, J.; Andersson, G.; Enmark, E.; Pettersson, K.; Warner, M.; Gustafsson, J. A., Mechanisms of estrogen action. *Physiol Rev* **2001,** 81, (4), 1535-65.

[77] Le Dily, F.; Beato, M., Signaling by Steroid Hormones in the 3D Nuclear Space. *Int J Mol Sci* **2018,** 19, (2).

[78] Andersen, J.; DyReyes, V. M.; Barbieri, R. L.; Coachman, D. M.; Miksicek, R. J., Leiomyoma primary cultures have elevated transcriptional response to estrogen compared with autologous myometrial cultures. *J Soc Gynecol Investig* **1995,** 2, (3), 542-51.

[79] Kim, J. J.; Kurita, T.; Bulun, S. E., Progesterone action in endometrial cancer, endometriosis, uterine fibroids, and breast cancer. *Endocr Rev* **2013,** 34, (1), 130-62.

[80] Stewart, E. A.; Friedman, A. J.; Peck, K.; Nowak, R. A., Relative overexpression of collagen type I and collagen type III messenger ribonucleic acids by uterine leiomyomas during the proliferative phase of the menstrual cycle. *J Clin Endocrinol Metab* **1994,** 79, (3), 900-6.

[81] Wei, J.; Chiriboga, L.; Mizuguchi, M.; Yee, H.; Mittal, K., Expression profile of tuberin and some potential tumorigenic factors in 60 patients with uterine leiomyomata. *Mod Pathol* **2005,** 18, (2), 179-88.

[82] Hassan, M. H.; Salama, S. A.; Arafa, H. M.; Hamada, F. M.; Al-Hendy, A., Adenovirus-mediated delivery of a dominant-negative estrogen receptor gene in uterine leiomyoma cells abrogates estrogen- and progesterone-regulated gene expression. *J Clin Endocrinol Metab* **2007,** 92, (10), 3949-57.

[83] Hassan, M. H.; Salama, S. A.; Zhang, D.; Arafa, H. M.; Hamada, F. M.; Fouad, H.; Walker, C. C.; Al-Hendy, A., Gene therapy targeting leiomyoma: adenovirus-mediated delivery of

dominant-negative estrogen receptor gene shrinks uterine tumors in Eker rat model. *Fertil Steril* **2010,** 93, (1), 239-50.

[84] Ciarmela, P.; Islam, M. S.; Reis, F. M.; Gray, P. C.; Bloise, E.; Petraglia, F.; Vale, W.; Castellucci, M., Growth factors and myometrium: biological effects in uterine fibroid and possible clinical implications. *Hum Reprod Update* **2011,** 17, (6), 772-90.

[85] Arici, A.; Sozen, I., Transforming growth factor-beta3 is expressed at high levels in leiomyoma where it stimulates fibronectin expression and cell proliferation. *Fertil Steril* **2000,** 73, (5), 1006-11.

[86] Inagaki, N.; Ung, L.; Otani, T.; Wilkinson, D.; Lopata, A., Uterine cavity matrix metalloproteinases and cytokines in patients with leiomyoma, adenomyosis or endometrial polyp. *Eur J Obstet Gynecol Reprod Biol* **2003,** 111, (2), 197-203.

[87] Protic, O.; Islam, M. S.; Greco, S.; Giannubilo, S. R.; Lamanna, P.; Petraglia, F.; Ciavattini, A.; Castellucci, M.; Hinz, B.; Ciarmela, P., Activin A in Inflammation, Tissue Repair, and Fibrosis: Possible Role as Inflammatory and Fibrotic Mediator of Uterine Fibroid Development and Growth. *Semin Reprod Med* **2017,** 35, (6), 499-509.

[88] Munger, J. S.; Sheppard, D., Cross talk among TGF-beta signaling pathways, integrins, and the extracellular matrix. *Cold Spring Harb Perspect Biol* **2011,** 3, (11), a005017.

[89] Baird, D. D.; Travlos, G.; Wilson, R.; Dunson, D. B.; Hill, M. C.; D'Aloisio, A. A.; London, S. J.; Schectman, J. M., Uterine leiomyomata in relation to insulin-like growth factor-I, insulin, and diabetes. *Epidemiology* **2009,** 20, (4), 604-10.

[90] Boehm, K. D.; Daimon, M.; Gorodeski, I. G.; Sheean, L. A.; Utian, W. H.; Ilan, J., Expression of the insulin-like and platelet-derived growth factor genes in human uterine tissues. *Mol Reprod Dev* **1990,** 27, (2), 93-101.

[91] Burroughs, K. D.; Howe, S. R.; Okubo, Y.; Fuchs-Young, R.; LeRoith, D.; Walker, C. L., Dysregulation of IGF-I signaling in uterine leiomyoma. *J Endocrinol* **2002,** 172, (1), 83-93.

[92] Swartz, C. D.; Afshari, C. A.; Yu, L.; Hall, K. E.; Dixon, D., Estrogen-induced changes in IGF-I, Myb family and MAP kinase pathway genes in human uterine leiomyoma and normal uterine smooth muscle cell lines. *Mol Hum Reprod* **2005,** 11, (6), 441-50.

[93] Friedman, A. J.; Rein, M. S.; Pandian, M. R.; Barbieri, R. L., Fasting serum growth hormone and insulin-like growth factor-I and -II concentrations in women with leiomyomata uteri treated with leuprolide acetate or placebo. *Fertil Steril* **1990,** 53, (2), 250-3.

[94] Englund, K.; Lindblom, B.; Carlstrom, K.; Gustavsson, I.; Sjoblom, P.; Blanck, A., Gene expression and tissue concentrations of IGF-I in human myometrium and fibroids under different hormonal conditions. *Mol Hum Reprod* **2000,** 6, (10), 915-20.

[95] Ono, M.; Yin, P.; Navarro, A.; Moravek, M. B.; Coon, J. S. t.; Druschitz, S. A.; Serna, V. A.; Qiang, W.; Brooks, D. C.; Malpani, S. S.; Ma, J.; Ercan, C. M.; Mittal, N.; Monsivais, D.; Dyson, M. T.; Yemelyanov, A.; Maruyama, T.; Chakravarti, D.; Kim, J. J.; Kurita, T.; Gottardi, C. J.; Bulun, S. E., Paracrine activation of WNT/beta-catenin pathway in uterine leiomyoma stem cells promotes tumor growth. *Proc Natl Acad Sci U S A* **2013,** 110, (42), 17053-8.

[96] Islam, M. S.; Catherino, W. H.; Protic, O.; Janjusevic, M.; Gray, P. C.; Giannubilo, S. R.; Ciavattini, A.; Lamanna, P.; Tranquilli, A. L.; Petraglia, F.; Castellucci, M.; Ciarmela, P., Role

of activin-A and myostatin and their signaling pathway in human myometrial and leiomyoma cell function. *J Clin Endocrinol Metab* **2014,** 99, (5), E775-85.

[97] Al-Hendy, A.; Laknaur, A.; Diamond, M. P.; Ismail, N.; Boyer, T. G.; Halder, S. K., Silencing Med12 Gene Reduces Proliferation of Human Leiomyoma Cells Mediated via Wnt/beta-Catenin Signaling Pathway. *Endocrinology* **2017,** 158, (3), 592-603.

[98] Donnez, J.; Dolmans, M. M., Uterine fibroid management: from the present to the future. *Hum Reprod Update* **2016,** 22, (6), 665-686.

[99] Cheng, Z.; Xie, Y.; Dai, H.; Hu, L.; Zhu, Y.; Gong, J., Unequal tissue expression of proteins from the PA/PAI system, myoma necrosis, and uterus survival after uterine artery occlusion. *Int J Gynaecol Obstet* **2008,** 102, (1), 55-9.

[100] Walker, C. L., Role of hormonal and reproductive factors in the etiology and treatment of uterine leiomyoma. *Recent Prog Horm Res* **2002,** 57, 277-94.

[101] El Andaloussi, A.; Al-Hendy, A.; Ismail, N.; Boyer, T. G.; Halder, S. K., Introduction of Somatic Mutation in MED12 Induces Wnt4/beta-Catenin and Disrupts Autophagy in Human Uterine Myometrial Cell. *Reprod Sci* **2020,** 27, (3), 823-832.

[102] Ali, M.; Shahin, S. M.; Sabri, N. A.; Al-Hendy, A.; Yang, Q., Activation of beta-Catenin Signaling and its Crosstalk With Estrogen and Histone Deacetylases in Human Uterine Fibroids. *J Clin Endocrinol Metab* **2020,** 105, (4).

[103] Lewis, T. D.; Malik, M.; Britten, J.; Parikh, T.; Cox, J.; Catherino, W. H., Ulipristal acetate decreases active TGF-beta3 and its canonical signaling in uterine leiomyoma via two novel mechanisms. *Fertil Steril* **2019,** 111, (4), 806-815 e1.

[104] Ono, M.; Yin, P.; Navarro, A.; Moravek, M. B.; Coon, V. J.; Druschitz, S. A.; Gottardi, C. J.; Bulun, S. E., Inhibition of canonical WNT signaling attenuates human leiomyoma cell growth. *Fertil Steril* **2014,** 101, (5), 1441-9.

[105] Garner, C., Uses of GnRH agonists. *Journal of obstetric, gynecologic, and neonatal nursing : JOGNN* **1994,** 23, (7), 563-70.

[106] Sabry, M.; Al-Hendy, A., Medical treatment of uterine leiomyoma. *Reproductive sciences* **2012,** 19, (4), 339-53.

[107] Al-Hendy, A.; Salama, S., Gene therapy and uterine leiomyoma: a review. *Human reproduction update* **2006,** 12, (4), 385-400.

[108] Zeng, L.; Yang, K.; Liu, H.; Zhang, G., A network pharmacology approach to investigate the pharmacological effects of Guizhi Fuling Wan on uterine fibroids. *Experimental and therapeutic medicine* **2017,** 14, (5), 4697-4710.

[109] Su, S. Y.; Muo, C. H.; Morisky, D. E., Use of chinese medicine and subsequent surgery in women with uterine fibroid: a retrospective cohort study. *Evidence-based complementary and alternative medicine : eCAM* **2012,** 2012, 617918.

[110] Ohara, N.; Morikawa, A.; Chen, W.; Wang, J.; DeManno, D. A.; Chwalisz, K.; Maruo, T., Comparative effects of SPRM asoprisnil (J867) on proliferation, apoptosis, and the expression of growth factors in cultured uterine leiomyoma cells and normal myometrial cells. *Reproductive sciences* **2007,** 14, (8 Suppl), 20-7.

[111] Hewlings, S. J.; Kalman, D. S., Curcumin: A Review of Its Effects on Human Health. *Foods* **2017,** 6, (10).

[112] Srivastava, R.; Dikshit, M.; Srimal, R. C.; Dhawan, B. N., Anti-thrombotic

effect of curcumin. *Thromb Res* **1985,** 40, (3), 413-7.

[113] Soudamini, K. K.; Unnikrishnan, M. C.; Soni, K. B.; Kuttan, R., Inhibition of lipid peroxidation and cholesterol levels in mice by curcumin. *Indian J Physiol Pharmacol* **1992,** 36, (4), 239-43.

[114] Asai, A.; Miyazawa, T., Dietary curcuminoids prevent high-fat diet-induced lipid accumulation in rat liver and epididymal adipose tissue. *J Nutr* **2001,** 131, (11), 2932-5.

[115] Venkatesan, N., Curcumin attenuation of acute adriamycin myocardial toxicity in rats. *Br J Pharmacol* **1998,** 124, (3), 425-7.

[116] Aggarwal, B. B.; Kumar, A.; Bharti, A. C., Anticancer potential of curcumin: preclinical and clinical studies. *Anticancer Res* **2003,** 23, (1A), 363-98.

[117] Mukhopadhyay, A.; Banerjee, S.; Stafford, L. J.; Xia, C.; Liu, M.; Aggarwal, B. B., Curcumin-induced suppression of cell proliferation correlates with down-regulation of cyclin D1 expression and CDK4-mediated retinoblastoma protein phosphorylation. *Oncogene* **2002,** 21, (57), 8852-61.

[118] Gupta, S. C.; Prasad, S.; Kim, J. H.; Patchva, S.; Webb, L. J.; Priyadarsini, I. K.; Aggarwal, B. B., Multitargeting by curcumin as revealed by molecular interaction studies. *Nat Prod Rep* **2011,** 28, (12), 1937-55.

[119] Anand, P.; Sundaram, C.; Jhurani, S.; Kunnumakkara, A. B.; Aggarwal, B. B., Curcumin and cancer: an "old-age" disease with an "age-old" solution. *Cancer Lett* **2008,** 267, (1), 133-64.

[120] Goel, A.; Kunnumakkara, A. B.; Aggarwal, B. B., Curcumin as "Curecumin": from kitchen to clinic. *Biochem Pharmacol* **2008,** 75, (4), 787-809.

[121] Kunnumakkara, A. B.; Anand, P.; Aggarwal, B. B., Curcumin inhibits proliferation, invasion, angiogenesis and metastasis of different cancers through interaction with multiple cell signaling proteins. *Cancer Lett* **2008,** 269, (2), 199-225.

[122] Sissener, N. H.; Johannessen, L. E.; Hevroy, E. M.; Wiik-Nielsen, C. R.; Berdal, K. G.; Nordgreen, A.; Hemre, G. I., Zebrafish (*Danio rerio*) as a model for investigating the safety of GM feed ingredients (soya and maize); performance, stress response and uptake of dietary DNA sequences. *Br J Nutr* **2010,** 103, (1), 3-15.

[123] Houston, K. D.; Copland, J. A.; Broaddus, R. R.; Gottardis, M. M.; Fischer, S. M.; Walker, C. L., Inhibition of proliferation and estrogen receptor signaling by peroxisome proliferator-activated receptor gamma ligands in uterine leiomyoma. *Cancer Res* **2003,** 63, (6), 1221-7.

[124] Lev-Ari, S.; Starr, A.; Vexler, A.; Karaush, V.; Loew, V.; Greif, J.; Fenig, E.; Aderka, D.; Ben-Yosef, R., Inhibition of pancreatic and lung adenocarcinoma cell survival by curcumin is associated with increased apoptosis, down-regulation of COX-2 and EGFR and inhibition of Erk1/2 activity. *Anticancer Res* **2006,** 26, (6B), 4423-30.

[125] Chen, X.; Chen, X.; Shi, X.; Gao, Z.; Guo, Z., Curcumin attenuates endothelial cell fibrosis through inhibiting endothelial-interstitial transformation. *Clin Exp Pharmacol Physiol* **2020,** 47, (7), 1182-1192.

[126] Bajracharya, P.; Lee, E. J.; Lee, D. M.; Shim, S. H.; Kim, K. J.; Lee, S. H.; Bae, J. J.; Chun, S. S.; Lee, T. K.; Kwon, S. H.; Choi, I., Effect of different ingredients in traditional Korean medicine for human uterine leiomyoma on normal myometrial and leiomyomal smooth muscle cell proliferation. *Arch Pharm Res* **2009,** 32, (11), 1555-63.

[127] Malik, M.; Mendoza, M.; Payson, M.; Catherino, W. H., Curcumin, a nutritional supplement with antineoplastic activity, enhances leiomyoma cell apoptosis and decreases fibronectin expression. *Fertil Steril* **2009,** 91, (5 Suppl), 2177-84.

[128] Wright, H. M.; Clish, C. B.; Mikami, T.; Hauser, S.; Yanagi, K.; Hiramatsu, R.; Serhan, C. N.; Spiegelman, B. M., A synthetic antagonist for the peroxisome proliferator-activated receptor gamma inhibits adipocyte differentiation. *J Biol Chem* **2000,** 275, (3), 1873-7.

[129] Sharma, A. M.; Staels, B., Review: Peroxisome proliferator-activated receptor gamma and adipose tissue--understanding obesity-related changes in regulation of lipid and glucose metabolism. *J Clin Endocrinol Metab* **2007,** 92, (2), 386-95.

[130] Chen, A.; Xu, J., Activation of PPAR{gamma} by curcumin inhibits Moser cell growth and mediates suppression of gene expression of cyclin D1 and EGFR. *Am J Physiol Gastrointest Liver Physiol* **2005,** 288, (3), G447-56.

[131] Takeda, T.; Sakata, M.; Isobe, A.; Miyake, A.; Nishimoto, F.; Ota, Y.; Kamiura, S.; Kimura, T., Relationship between metabolic syndrome and uterine leiomyomas: a case-control study. *Gynecol Obstet Invest* **2008,** 66, (1), 14-7.

[132] Tsuiji, K.; Takeda, T.; Li, B.; Wakabayashi, A.; Kondo, A.; Kimura, T.; Yaegashi, N., Inhibitory effect of curcumin on uterine leiomyoma cell proliferation. *Gynecol Endocrinol* **2011,** 27, (7), 512-7.

[133] Wahlstrom, B.; Blennow, G., A study on the fate of curcumin in the rat. *Acta Pharmacol Toxicol (Copenh)* **1978,** 43, (2), 86-92.

[134] Ravindranath, V.; Chandrasekhara, N., Absorption and tissue distribution of curcumin in rats. *Toxicology* **1980,** 16, (3), 259-65.

[135] Shoba, G.; Joy, D.; Joseph, T.; Majeed, M.; Rajendran, R.; Srinivas, P. S., Influence of piperine on the pharmacokinetics of curcumin in animals and human volunteers. *Planta Med* **1998,** 64, (4), 353-6.

[136] Pan, M. H.; Huang, T. M.; Lin, J. K., Biotransformation of curcumin through reduction and glucuronidation in mice. *Drug Metab Dispos* **1999,** 27, (4), 486-94.

[137] Cen, L.; Hutzen, B.; Ball, S.; DeAngelis, S.; Chen, C. L.; Fuchs, J. R.; Li, C.; Li, P. K.; Lin, J., New structural analogues of curcumin exhibit potent growth suppressive activity in human colorectal carcinoma cells. *BMC Cancer* **2009,** 9, 99.

[138] Shibata, H.; Yamakoshi, H.; Sato, A.; Ohori, H.; Kakudo, Y.; Kudo, C.; Takahashi, Y.; Watanabe, M.; Takano, H.; Ishioka, C.; Noda, T.; Iwabuchi, Y., Newly synthesized curcumin analog has improved potential to prevent colorectal carcinogenesis in vivo. *Cancer Sci* **2009,** 100, (5), 956-60.

[139] Costa, C.; Tsatsakis, A.; Mamoulakis, C.; Teodoro, M.; Briguglio, G.; Caruso, E.; Tsoukalas, D.; Margina, D.; Dardiotis, E.; Kouretas, D.; Fenga, C., Current evidence on the effect of dietary polyphenols intake on chronic diseases. *Food and chemical toxicology: an international journal published for the British Industrial Biological Research Association* **2017,** 110, 286-299.

[140] Banerjee, S.; Bueso-Ramos, C.; Aggarwal, B. B., Suppression of 7,12-dimethylbenz(a)anthracene-induced mammary carcinogenesis in rats by resveratrol: role of nuclear factor-kappaB, cyclooxygenase 2, and matrix metalloprotease 9. *Cancer research* **2002,** 62, (17), 4945-54.

[141] Jang, M.; Cai, L.; Udeani, G. O.; Slowing, K. V.; Thomas, C. F.; Beecher, C. W.; Fong, H. H.; Farnsworth, N. R.; Kinghorn, A. D.; Mehta, R. G.; Moon, R. C.; Pezzuto, J. M., Cancer chemopreventive activity of resveratrol, a natural product derived from grapes. *Science* **1997,** 275, (5297), 218-20.

[142] Lin, H. Y.; Hsieh, M. T.; Cheng, G. Y.; Lai, H. Y.; Chin, Y. T.; Shih, Y. J.; Nana, A. W.; Lin, S. Y.; Yang, Y. S. H.; Tang, H. Y.; Chiang, I. J.; Wang, K., Mechanisms of action of nonpeptide hormones on resveratrol-induced antiproliferation of cancer cells. *Annals of the New York Academy of Sciences* **2017,** 1403, (1), 92-100.

[143] Ho, Y.; Lin, Y. S.; Liu, H. L.; Shih, Y. J.; Lin, S. Y.; Shih, A.; Chin, Y. T.; Chen, Y. R.; Lin, H. Y.; Davis, P. J., Biological Mechanisms by Which Antiproliferative Actions of Resveratrol Are Minimized. *Nutrients* **2017,** 9, (10).

[144] Cheng, T. M.; Chin, Y. T.; Ho, Y.; Chen, Y. R.; Yang, Y. N.; Yang, Y. C.; Shih, Y. J.; Lin, T. I.; Lin, H. Y.; Davis, P. J., Resveratrol induces sumoylated COX-2-dependent anti-proliferation in human prostate cancer LNCaP cells. *Food and chemical toxicology : an international journal published for the British Industrial Biological Research Association* **2017,** 112, 67-75.

[145] Chin, Y. T.; Yang, S. H.; Chang, T. C.; Changou, C. A.; Lai, H. Y.; Fu, E.; HuangFu, W. C.; Davis, P. J.; Lin, H. Y.; Liu, L. F., Mechanisms of dihydrotestosterone action on resveratrol-induced anti-proliferation in breast cancer cells with different ERalpha status. *Oncotarget* **2015,** 6, (34), 35866-79.

[146] Chow, S. E.; Wang, J. S.; Chuang, S. F.; Chang, Y. L.; Chu, W. K.; Chen, W. S.; Chen, Y. W., Resveratrol-induced p53-independent apoptosis of human nasopharyngeal carcinoma cells is correlated with the downregulation of DeltaNp63. *Cancer Gene Ther* **2010,** 17, (12), 872-82.

[147] Schmidt, A. H.; Solloch, U. V.; Pingel, J.; Sauter, J.; Bohme, I.; Cereb, N.; Dubicka, K.; Schumacher, S.; Wachowiak, J.; Ehninger, G., Regional HLA differences in Poland and their effect on stem cell donor registry planning. *PLoS One* **2013,** 8, (9), e73835.

[148] Rasheduzzaman, M.; Jeong, J. K.; Park, S. Y., Resveratrol sensitizes lung cancer cell to TRAIL by p53 independent and suppression of Akt/NF-kappaB signaling. *Life Sci* **2018,** 208, 208-220.

[149] Alamolhodaei, N. S.; Tsatsakis, A. M.; Ramezani, M.; Hayes, A. W.; Karimi, G., Resveratrol as MDR reversion molecule in breast cancer: An overview. *Food and chemical toxicology: an international journal published for the British Industrial Biological Research Association* **2017,** 103, 223-232.

[150] Turner, R. S.; Thomas, R. G.; Craft, S.; van Dyck, C. H.; Mintzer, J.; Reynolds, B. A.; Brewer, J. B.; Rissman, R. A.; Raman, R.; Aisen, P. S.; Alzheimer's Disease Cooperative, S., A randomized, double-blind, placebo-controlled trial of resveratrol for Alzheimer disease. *Neurology* **2015,** 85, (16), 1383-91.

[151] Chin, Y. T.; Hsieh, M. T.; Lin, C. Y.; Kuo, P. J.; Yang, Y. C.; Shih, Y. J.; Lai, H. Y.; Cheng, G. Y.; Tang, H. Y.; Lee, C. C.; Lee, S. Y.; Wang, C. C.; Lin, H. Y.; Fu, E.; Whang-Peng, J.; Liu, L. F., 2,3,5,4'-Tetrahydroxystilbene-2-O-beta-glucoside Isolated from Polygoni Multiflori Ameliorates the Development of Periodontitis. *Mediators Inflamm* **2016,** 2016, 6953459.

[152] Riaz, A.; Ilan, N.; Vlodavsky, I.; Li, J. P.; Johansson, S., Characterization of heparanase-induced phosphatidylinositol 3-kinase-AKT activation and its integrin dependence. *J Biol Chem* **2013,** 288, (17), 12366-75.

[153] Nakajima, S.; Ishimaru, K.; Kobayashi, A.; Yu, G.; Nakamura, Y.; Oh-Oka, K.; Suzuki-Inoue, K.; Kono, K.; Nakao, A., Resveratrol inhibits IL-33-mediated mast cell activation by targeting the MK2/3-PI3K/Akt axis. *Sci Rep* **2019,** 9, (1), 18423.

[154] Lin, H. Y.; Chin, Y. T.; Yang, Y. C.; Lai, H. Y.; Wang-Peng, J.; Liu, L. F.; Tang, H. Y.; Davis, P. J., Thyroid Hormone, Cancer, and Apoptosis. *Compr Physiol* **2016,** 6, (3), 1221-37.

[155] Davis, P. J.; Lin, H. Y.; Hercbergs, A.; Keating, K. A.; Mousa, S. A., Coronaviruses and Integrin alphavbeta3: Does Thyroid Hormone Modify the Relationship? *Endocr Res* **2020,** 45, (3), 210-215.

[156] Zaidel-Bar, R.; Itzkovitz, S.; Ma'ayan, A.; Iyengar, R.; Geiger, B., Functional atlas of the integrin adhesome. *Nat Cell Biol* **2007,** 9, (8), 858-67.

[157] Zaidel-Bar, R.; Geiger, B., The switchable integrin adhesome. *J Cell Sci* **2010,** 123, (Pt 9), 1385-8.

[158] Huveneers, S.; Danen, E. H., Adhesion signaling - crosstalk between integrins, Src and Rho. *J Cell Sci* **2009,** 122, (Pt 8), 1059-69.

[159] Streuli, C. H.; Akhtar, N., Signal co-operation between integrins and other receptor systems. *Biochem J* **2009,** 418, (3), 491-506.

[160] Ivaska, J.; Heino, J., Interplay between cell adhesion and growth factor receptors: from the plasma membrane to the endosomes. *Cell Tissue Res* **2010,** 339, (1), 111-20.

[161] Arslan, A. A.; Gold, L. I.; Mittal, K.; Suen, T. C.; Belitskaya-Levy, I.; Tang, M. S.; Toniolo, P., Gene expression studies provide clues to the pathogenesis of uterine leiomyoma: new evidence and a systematic review. *Hum Reprod* **2005,** 20, (4), 852-63.

[162] Ock, S.; Ahn, J.; Lee, S. H.; Kang, H.; Offermanns, S.; Ahn, H. Y.; Jo, Y. S.; Shong, M.; Cho, B. Y.; Jo, D.; Abel, E. D.; Lee, T. J.; Park, W. J.; Lee, I. K.; Kim, J., IGF-1 receptor deficiency in thyrocytes impairs thyroid hormone secretion and completely inhibits TSH-stimulated goiter. *FASEB J* **2013,** 27, (12), 4899-908.

[163] Hong Bin, W.; Da, L. H.; Xue, Y.; Jing, B., Pterostilbene (3′,5′-dimethoxy-resveratrol) exerts potent antitumor effects in HeLa human cervical cancer cells via disruption of mitochondrial membrane potential, apoptosis induction and targeting m-TOR/PI3K/Akt signalling pathway. *J BUON* **2018,** 23, (5), 1384-1389.

[164] Vanamala, J.; Reddivari, L.; Radhakrishnan, S.; Tarver, C., Resveratrol suppresses IGF-1 induced human colon cancer cell proliferation and elevates apoptosis via suppression of IGF-1R/Wnt and activation of p53 signaling pathways. *BMC Cancer* **2010,** 10, 238.

[165] Gionfra, F.; De Vito, P.; Pallottini, V.; Lin, H. Y.; Davis, P. J.; Pedersen, J. Z.; Incerpi, S., The Role of Thyroid Hormones in Hepatocyte Proliferation and Liver Cancer. *Front Endocrinol (Lausanne)* **2019,** 10, 532.

[166] Kim, K. H.; Back, J. H.; Zhu, Y.; Arbesman, J.; Athar, M.; Kopelovich, L.; Kim, A. L.; Bickers, D. R., Resveratrol targets transforming growth factor-beta2 signaling to block UV-induced tumor progression. *J Invest Dermatol* **2011,** 131, (1), 195-202.

[167] Sexton, E.; Van Themsche, C.; LeBlanc, K.; Parent, S.; Lemoine, P.; Asselin, E., Resveratrol interferes with AKT activity and triggers apoptosis in human uterine cancer cells. *Mol Cancer* **2006,** 5, 45.

[168] Tanwar, P. S.; Lee, H. J.; Zhang, L.; Zukerberg, L. R.; Taketo, M. M.; Rueda, B. R.; Teixeira, J. M., Constitutive

activation of Beta-catenin in uterine stroma and smooth muscle leads to the development of mesenchymal tumors in mice. *Biol Reprod* **2009,** 81, (3), 545-52.

[169] Ko, Y. A.; Jamaluddin, M. F. B.; Adebayo, M.; Bajwa, P.; Scott, R. J.; Dharmarajan, A. M.; Nahar, P.; Tanwar, P. S., Extracellular matrix (ECM) activates beta-catenin signaling in uterine fibroids. *Reproduction* **2018,** 155, (1), 61-71.

[170] Nana, A. W.; Chin, Y. T.; Lin, C. Y.; Ho, Y.; Bennett, J. A.; Shih, Y. J.; Chen, Y. R.; Changou, C. A.; Pedersen, J. Z.; Incerpi, S.; Liu, L. F.; Whang-Peng, J.; Fu, E.; Li, W. S.; Mousa, S. A.; Lin, H. Y.; Davis, P. J., Tetrac downregulates beta-catenin and HMGA2 to promote the effect of resveratrol in colon cancer. *Endocr Relat Cancer* **2018,** 25, (3), 279-293.

[171] Lee, Y. S.; Chin, Y. T.; Shih, Y. J.; Nana, A. W.; Chen, Y. R.; Wu, H. C.; Yang, Y. S. H.; Lin, H. Y.; Davis, P. J., Thyroid Hormone Promotes beta-Catenin Activation and Cell Proliferation in Colorectal Cancer. *Horm Cancer* **2018,** 9, (3), 156-165.

[172] Lin, H. Y.; Delmas, D.; Vang, O.; Hsieh, T. C.; Lin, S.; Cheng, G. Y.; Chiang, H. L.; Chen, C. E.; Tang, H. Y.; Crawford, D. R.; Whang-Peng, J.; Hwang, J.; Liu, L. F.; Wu, J. M., Mechanisms of ceramide-induced COX-2-dependent apoptosis in human ovarian cancer OVCAR-3 cells partially overlapped with resveratrol. *J Cell Biochem* **2013,** 114, (8), 1940-54.

[173] Chin, Y. T.; Wei, P. L.; Ho, Y.; Nana, A. W.; Changou, C. A.; Chen, Y. R.; Yang, Y. S.; Hsieh, M. T.; Hercbergs, A.; Davis, P. J.; Shih, Y. J.; Lin, H. Y., Thyroxine inhibits resveratrol-caused apoptosis by PD-L1 in ovarian cancer cells. *Endocr Relat Cancer* **2018,** 25, (5), 533-545.

[174] Kim, D. I.; Lee, T. K.; Lim, I. S.; Kim, H.; Lee, Y. C.; Kim, C. H., Regulation of IGF-I production and proliferation of human leiomyomal smooth muscle cells by Scutellaria barbata D. Don in vitro: isolation of flavonoids of apigenin and luteolin as acting compounds. *Toxicol Appl Pharmacol* **2005,** 205, (3), 213-24.

[175] Lee, T. K.; Lee, D. K.; Kim, D. I.; Lee, Y. C.; Chang, Y. C.; Kim, C. H., Inhibitory effects of Scutellaria barbata D. Don on human uterine leiomyomal smooth muscle cell proliferation through cell cycle analysis. *Int Immunopharmacol* **2004,** 4, (3), 447-54.

[176] Zhang, S.; Cao, H. J.; Davis, F. B.; Tang, H. Y.; Davis, P. J.; Lin, H. Y., Oestrogen inhibits resveratrol-induced post-translational modification of p53 and apoptosis in breast cancer cells. *Br J Cancer* **2004,** 91, (1), 178-85.

[177] Hu, C.; Liu, Y.; Teng, M.; Jiao, K.; Zhen, J.; Wu, M.; Li, Z., Resveratrol inhibits the proliferation of estrogen receptor-positive breast cancer cells by suppressing EZH2 through the modulation of ERK1/2 signaling. *Cell Biol Toxicol* **2019,** 35, (5), 445-456.

[178] Chao, A.; Lin, C. Y.; Tsai, C. L.; Hsueh, S.; Lin, Y. Y.; Lin, C. T.; Chou, H. H.; Wang, T. H.; Lai, C. H.; Wang, H. S., Estrogen stimulates the proliferation of human endometrial cancer cells by stabilizing nucleophosmin/B23 (NPM/B23). *J Mol Med (Berl)* **2013,** 91, (2), 249-59.

[179] Sun, Y.; Wang, C.; Yang, H.; Ma, X., The effect of estrogen on the proliferation of endometrial cancer cells is mediated by ERRgamma through AKT and ERK1/2. *Eur J Cancer Prev* **2014,** 23, (5), 418-24.

[180] Jiang, X.; Ye, X.; Ma, J.; Li, W.; Wu, R.; Jun, L., G protein-coupled estrogen receptor 1 (GPER 1) mediates

estrogen-induced, proliferation of leiomyoma cells. *Gynecol Endocrinol* **2015,** 31, (11), 894-8.

[181] Cheng, T. M.; Chin, Y. T.; Ho, Y.; Chen, Y. R.; Yang, Y. N.; Yang, Y. C.; Shih, Y. J.; Lin, T. I.; Lin, H. Y.; Davis, P. J., Resveratrol induces sumoylated COX-2-dependent anti-proliferation in human prostate cancer LNCaP cells. *Food Chem Toxicol* **2018,** 112, 67-75.

[182] Parinandi, N. L.; Maulik, N.; Thirunavukkarasu, M.; McFadden, D. W., Antioxidants in Longevity and Medicine 2014. *Oxid Med Cell Longev* **2015,** 2015, 739417.

[183] Zhang, S. H.; Wang, W. Q.; Wang, J. L., Protective effect of tetrahydroxystilbene glucoside on cardiotoxicity induced by doxorubicin in vitro and in vivo. *Acta Pharmacol Sin* **2009,** 30, (11), 1479-87.

[184] Zhao, Y. Y.; Zhang, L.; Feng, Y. L.; Chen, D. Q.; Xi, Z. H.; Du, X.; Bai, X.; Lin, R. C., Pharmacokinetics of 2,3,5,4′-tetrahydroxystilbene-2-O-beta-D-glucoside in rat using ultra-performance LC-quadrupole TOF-MS. *J Sep Sci* **2013,** 36, (5), 863-71.

[185] Liu, Q. L.; Xiao, J. H.; Ma, R.; Ban, Y.; Wang, J. L., Effect of 2,3,5,4′-tetrahydroxystilbene-2-O-beta-D-glucoside on lipoprotein oxidation and proliferation of coronary arterial smooth cells. *J Asian Nat Prod Res* **2007,** 9, (6-8), 689-97.

[186] Li, F.; Zhang, T.; He, Y.; Gu, W.; Yang, X.; Zhao, R.; Yu, J., Inflammation inhibition and gut microbiota regulation by TSG to combat atherosclerosis in ApoE(-/-) mice. *J Ethnopharmacol* **2020,** 247, 112232.

[187] Wang, T.; Gu, J.; Wu, P. F.; Wang, F.; Xiong, Z.; Yang, Y. J.; Wu, W. N.; Dong, L. D.; Chen, J. G., Protection by tetrahydroxystilbene glucoside against cerebral ischemia: involvement of JNK, SIRT1, and NF-kappaB pathways and inhibition of intracellular ROS/RNS generation. *Free Radic Biol Med* **2009,** 47, (3), 229-40.

[188] Zhang, Y. Z.; Shen, J. F.; Xu, J. Y.; Xiao, J. H.; Wang, J. L., Inhibitory effects of 2,3,5,4′-tetrahydroxystilbene-2-O-beta-D-glucoside on experimental inflammation and cyclooxygenase 2 activity. *J Asian Nat Prod Res* **2007,** 9, (3-5), 355-63.

[189] D'Andrea, G., Pycnogenol: a blend of procyanidins with multifaceted therapeutic applications? *Fitoterapia* **2010,** 81, (7), 724-36.

[190] Petrassi, C.; Mastromarino, A.; Spartera, C., PYCNOGENOL in chronic venous insufficiency. *Phytomedicine* **2000,** 7, (5), 383-8.

[191] Ho, Y.; Chen, Y. F.; Wang, L. H.; Hsu, K. Y.; Chin, Y. T.; Yang, Y. S. H.; Wang, S. H.; Chen, Y. R.; Shih, Y. J.; Liu, L. F.; Wang, K.; Whang-Peng, J.; Tang, H. Y.; Lin, H. Y.; Liu, H. L.; Lin, S. J., Inhibitory Effect of Anoectochilus formosanus Extract on Hyperglycemia-Related PD-L1 Expression and Cancer Proliferation. *Front Pharmacol* **2018,** 9, 807.

[192] Ahmad, N.; Gupta, S.; Mukhtar, H., Green tea polyphenol epigallocatechin-3-gallate differentially modulates nuclear factor kappaB in cancer cells versus normal cells. *Arch Biochem Biophys* **2000,** 376, (2), 338-46.

[193] Beck, S. E.; Jung, B. H.; Fiorino, A.; Gomez, J.; Rosario, E. D.; Cabrera, B. L.; Huang, S. C.; Chow, J. Y.; Carethers, J. M., Bone morphogenetic protein signaling and growth suppression in colon cancer. *Am J Physiol Gastrointest Liver Physiol* **2006,** 291, (1), G135-45.

[194] Ahmed, R. S.; Liu, G.; Renzetti, A.; Farshi, P.; Yang, H.; Soave, C.; Saed, G.; El-Ghoneimy, A. A.; El-Banna, H. A.; Foldes, R.; Chan, T. H.; Dou, Q. P.,

Biological and Mechanistic Characterization of Novel Prodrugs of Green Tea Polyphenol Epigallocatechin Gallate Analogs in Human Leiomyoma Cell Lines. *J Cell Biochem* **2016,** 117, (10), 2357-69.

[195] Beltz, L. A.; Bayer, D. K.; Moss, A. L.; Simet, I. M., Mechanisms of cancer prevention by green and black tea polyphenols. *Anticancer Agents Med Chem* **2006,** 6, (5), 389-406.

[196] Kuhnel, F.; Zender, L.; Paul, Y.; Tietze, M. K.; Trautwein, C.; Manns, M.; Kubicka, S., NFkappaB mediates apoptosis through transcriptional activation of Fas (CD95) in adenoviral hepatitis. *J Biol Chem* **2000,** 275, (9), 6421-7.

[197] Maldonado, V.; Melendez-Zajgla, J.; Ortega, A., Modulation of NF-kappa B, and Bcl-2 in apoptosis induced by cisplatin in HeLa cells. *Mutat Res* **1997,** 381, (1), 67-75.

[198] Ahmad, N.; Cheng, P.; Mukhtar, H., Cell cycle dysregulation by green tea polyphenol epigallocatechin-3-gallate. *Biochem Biophys Res Commun* **2000,** 275, (2), 328-34.

[199] Nana, A. W.; Wu, S. Y.; Yang, Y. S.; Chin, Y. T.; Cheng, T. M.; Ho, Y.; Li, W. S.; Liao, Y. M.; Chen, Y. R.; Shih, Y. J.; Liu, Y. R.; Pedersen, J.; Incerpi, S.; Hercbergs, A.; Liu, L. F.; Whang-Peng, J.; Davis, P. J.; Lin, H. Y., Nano-Diamino-Tetrac (NDAT) Enhances Resveratrol-Induced Antiproliferation by Action on the RRM2 Pathway in Colorectal Cancers. *Horm Cancer* **2018,** 9, (5), 349-360.

Chapter 9

Perspective of Women about Her Body after Hysterectomy

Eman Alshawish

Abstract

Hysterectomy is the most common major gynecological operation in worldwide and Arabic countries. However, the psychological, physical and sexual consequences of hysterectomy are conflicting and the findings are mixed. While, some studies report that patients have experience greater improvement in their mental health, sexual desire and overall satisfaction. Others show that patients report various negative outcomes, with detrimental effects on sexual functioning being the main concern. My previous study demonstrated that hysterectomy had significantly negative effects on patients' body image, self-esteem, and identified common meanings and themes associated with hysterectomy stressors, which includes difficulties or limitations in physical and psychological aspects perceived by patients after hysterectomy. In this chapter, author will expand that discuss in details the different factors that influence the perspective of women about body after hysterectomy. Mainly, author will focus on religious, cultural, and psycho-social aspects. All of these factors are interacting with health status of women and effect the situation and productivity of women in her family and culture. Different strategy need to be adopted in order to overcome this problem using evidence and analysis of our Arabic culture and structure. Recommendation of study to health care profession as physician, nurses, midwives and other health care provider to be aware of these potential problematic issues in order to provide a competent health care for women based of her needs.

Keywords: fibroid, women's perception, hysterectomy, sexuality, self-esteem, body image, quality of life

1. Introduction and background

One in three women at age of 60 years in the USA have undergone a hysterectomy, it is the second most common major surgical procedure performed in women worldwide [1]. Also, it is the leading reason for non-obstetric surgery among women in many high-income settings [2–4]. Fibroids, dysfunctional uterine bleeding, uterine prolapse and chronic pelvic pain are the most indication for this surgery [5]. So, the majority of hysterectomies are performed on benign indications to improve quality of life with few complications post-operative.

In recent years, an increasing number of studies have shown long-term adverse effects of hysterectomy on the pelvic floor and some studies have demonstrated unwanted effects on other health aspects. Long-term effects of hysterectomy on the pelvic floor that should be considered in surgical decision making are: pelvic organ prolapse, urinary incontinence, bowel dysfunction, sexual function and pelvic organ fistula formation. These outcomes are particularly relevant as life expectancy

IntechOpen

has increased and sequel may occur a long time after the surgical procedure and severely [1]. The surgery can take an emotional toll on woman as well. These effects might be very personal; she may feel differently than others, this leads her to depression. Losing the ability to become pregnant is hard for many women in worldwide and especially in Arabic countries, where the reproductively in considered the main reason for marriage. Some women feel "changed." They may also mourn the loss of their fertility [6]. Fears of looking less "womanly" Younger women who have a hysterectomy sometimes are anxious about whether the surgery will change their appearance. They worry that it will make them more masculine [6]. A lot of Women who are the power of the community depressed, as a result of this operation, because of losing a something that a part of her femininity, make their body image and self-esteem disrupted, feelings that their different from others women who can childbearing, and she is not, all of that make them isolated from the community, when this community need for their power and productivity. In next section authors will highlighted on women perspective on her body, and focus on factors that might directly and indirectly influence these perspectives that includes religious, cultural, economic, political and psycho-social aspects based on review.

2. Narrative review

In this part, author will offer a narrative review that present a group of studies, to see the experiences and results of previous studies that discuss the experience of women who had done hysterectomy. As well as discuss the role of health care profession and recommended strategies to overcome these problem. This section will include four themes which are quality of life; physical and psychological changes; sexuality; Cultural and religious aspects; finally the review conclusion and recommendations.

Sexuality is written as separate theme not under physical and psychological theme due to its important and effects based on Maslow hierarchy. Another point is the sensitivity of talking in this subject in conservative Arabic culture even from health care profession themselves. If I ask myself if any of health care profession provided women with health education about her sexuality after hysterectomy, the answer is obviously clear. Might be there is no time to provide that after operation but the important point the negligence of this type of education. This indicates that health care professions are playing a big role to solve or complicate this issue. They have to deliver a competent health care for women based of her needs. This is the woman's right not luxury, especially for ethnic minorities group.

2.1 Quality of life

Improvements of quality of life and decrease gynecologic symptoms are the main reason of any decision that taken by women for undergoes hysterectomy. In a systematic review study, authors investigated and analyzed six studies which evaluated QOL after hysterectomy. The authors concluded that a significant improvement above baseline in QOL scores [7]. However, many evidence as illustrated in this review showed the suffer of women physically and psychologically post-operative.

Hysterectomy is the one of surgery that needs more physical & psychological support by nurses in hospitals or/and outpatient clinics. Also provide a full background or knowledge for women who will do a hysterectomy that help to avoid the impact of hysterectomy [8]. There are four major subjects relating to the participant's experience were identified by Valerie Fleming [9], doubts and justifications, pain, embodiment and sense of bitterness. In addition there are three domains must to integrate biophysical care of women, psychological, sociological, and spiritual domains [10]. Both of these study spotlight on the importance of provider training and education, also efforts must be directed to the community to enlighten men and families about hysterectomy by dispelling myths and providing current health information related to women's gynecological health and alternatives to, indications for, and types of hysterectomy.

2.2 Physical and psychological changes

As a result of study that examined by Gul Pinar et al., there is a relationships between hysterectomy and body image, self-esteem, and dyadic adjustment, which appears significantly in the scores, lower than the healthy women [11]. This indicates for the reduction of psychological support from community in general and family in specific. The most impact of hysterectomy as discussed on previous study [12], is the emotional side, seven themes that divided from this side, fear; pain; death and dying; numbness or delay in emotional reaction; bonding with baby; communication; and the need for information. Something that must to focus on managing it by enhances the quality of life or to avoid it before happened by providing correct health information by care providers. Like study which discussed in relation to the importance of information provision by gynecologists and its effects on women's decision-making about hysterectomy [13]. So gynecologists must initiate a comprehensive discussion about other treatments and their advantages and disadvantages. To explain the differences in complications between women after surgery, there are factors can determine this complication, Lifestyle factors (smoking and body mass index) and co-morbidity status, occupation and educational level [14].

The patients need for expressed their emotions and feelings after the major event that had happened in their life, otherwise, physical and psychological changes might be exaggerated. In previous qualitative study on Palestinian women, the most physical changes occur after hysterectomies were including pain, insomnia, eating disorder and immobility. One of the participants described pain as saying: *"I had never felt like this pain in my life"*. As a consequence of the pain, patients also suffer disturbances at night and changes in the sleep cycle. Also, Changes in the patients' appetite were reported in this study and it differs from one woman to another. Some of the participants expressed that their appetite increased and others reported the opposite. Another problem that reported was the immobility which affected the daily performance and routine activities at home [15].

Depression, accompanied by anxiety, de-socialization, and aggression, is the most common complication that reported by women after hysterectomy. The depression was figure as the most common psychological complication of hysterectomy [15, 16].

Also psychological and emotional stress was evident in previous study and shown a negative emotional outcome after hysterectomy. It has been suggested that early detection and immediate action by healthcare providers may prevent these negative impacts on the psychological wellbeing of these women. This is especially so in younger women in whom the psychological impacts are the greatest. Furthermore, because the main reason for the psychological impact was related to the immediate postmenopausal status after surgery, younger women appear to be more vulnerable, thus emphasizing the need for proper counseling in younger women undergoing hysterectomy [17].

The most coping mechanism and adaptation technique that used by women after operation from literature were praying, the Holy Quran, music, and other activities such as walking, sports (yoga) [15]. While, other study found that the operation affects patients' emotional reactions. As a result, they used these techniques to cope with their new condition and accept it [17].

2.3 Cultural and religious aspects

Another issue that should be highlighted in this review is the role and effect of environment as cultural and religious on the perception of women who undergo hysterectomy. The woman is not presented on isolation; she interacted with surrounding that affect her status and view to her body and problem. It is important to figure that uterus is representing woman's femininity and fertility.

The woman is not totally responsible for her body from legal and cultural aspect, it is partially. In Arabic countries as in Saudi Arabia and Palestine the health care system ask the husband's consent for any medical procedure that affects the reproductive ability of his wife. In recent study that disuses this practice in Saudi Arabia, author recommended that "arguments advocating for discontinuing the requirement are offered along with measures to implement in order to overcome this social artifact" [18].

However, Islamic law closely regulates and governs the life of every Muslim. The basic principle is that it is impermissible for a woman to have her uterus removed because this entails permanent sterilization, and this conflicts with one of the most important higher objectives of the Sharee'ah – fruitfulness in procreation. Anas ibn Maalik narrated that the Prophet, sallallaahu 'alayhi wa sallam, said: "Marry fertile affectionate women, for I will be proud of your numbers in front of the Prophets on the Day of Judgment." [19].

However, if there is concern of real or prevalent harm to the woman's health if the uterus is not removed, or it is feared that it could cause her death or bring about considerable hardship beyond her ability to endure, and it is necessary, according to the advice of reliable and experienced doctors, for the uterus to be removed to ward off such harm, then it is permissible for the woman to have her uterus removed. This is based on the well-established principles that "elimination of harm takes precedence to realization of benefit" and "necessity makes something prohibited permissible". Allaah The Exalted says (what means): {...while He has explained in detail to you what He has forbidden you, excepting that to which you are compelled.} [Quran 6:119].

Moreover, the Prophet, sallallaahu 'alayhi wa sallam, said: "There shall be no harm or reciprocal harm." [Musnad Ahmad and Al-Muwatta'] [19]. According to catholic a hysterectomy by choice over medical necessity would be a sin because it would cause permanent sterilization.

It is obviously clear here the gap between the cultural practice and religions aspect, what presented in religion in not translate totally to reality and practice. The women should have the total freedom to decide what she wants on her body. The powering women and taking her responsibilities will help her to cope well and accept any change to her body and soul.

From literature, other culture as presented in Indian, the author found the term "normalization of hysterectomy" was mentioned in many studies. The women are preferred to do hysterectomy as treatment for any menstrual or uterine problem instead of receiving medical or pharmacological treatment. This term underscores "the complex negotiations between women's agency and medically un indicated procedures, as well as the ethical obligations of providers—both of which require further consideration in the Indian context" [20]. However, this term is not presented in Arabic context; in contrast the family likes to have more children as highlighted above from religious and cultural side. Arabic families like to have more male children because they considered that in Arabic term "Ozwa" as a positive point and they will help them in future when parents become old. The more male children the women have delivered the more respect will receive from their culture, husband family and mother in law. So, we can imagine the scope of problem, how the effect of remove part of her women body "uterus" on her self-image.

2.4 Impact on sexual life

It is recognized that effects of hysterectomy on women's sexuality are debated and controversial from literature [17]. A Socio-cultural construction is main factor that influenced the sexuality that involves many factors such as gender, identity, sexual orientation, pleasure, intimacy, and reproduction [22]. Many previous studies reported that the majority of women and their partners reported zero negative impact on sexual satisfaction after abdominal hysterectomy, regardless of the surgery was subtotal or total to [23], for example the majority of Norwegian women and their partners reported no negative impact on sexual satisfaction after abdominal hysterectomy, regardless of whether the hysterectomy was subtotal or total [23]. While From the literature, some of the studies are inconsistent with these findings [15, 21–26, 35].

Other study reported that only one fourth of the women reported decreased sexual arousal, while the majority had experienced higher sexual arousal after abdominal and vaginal hysterectomy [27]. Various measures are used in these studies so comparing the degree of improvement in sexual is difficult. Guliz et al. mentioned in his study that advanced age, women's attitude towards sexuality, and type of hysterectomy are the main elements that determine sexual functioning after hysterectomy. Depression has a negative effect on sexual functioning [28]. A negative sexual experience before hysterectomy will be a strong predictor of having a negative sexual experience of partners after operation [23]. A survey conducted in Jordan, which is one of Arab countries found that sexual performance after hysterectomy was their most significant concern, and there was a significant improvement in sexual function for women undergoing this procedure [26].

When looking to change in sexual changes, Literature review reveals that dyspareunia, and a change in orgasm and/or less sex are happened to approximately 10 to 20% of the women who underwent a hysterectomy [29], and in post operatively sexual dysfunction [30–33], then after two years of operation the sexual dysfunction stabilized [24]. The main reason for sexual annoyances were included the modified self-image perception after surgery and decrease in vaginal lubrication a [34].

One of study revealed the negative impact of hysterectomy on the sexual life, which lead to increased depression and anxiety, with sexual dissatisfaction [35]. The counseling and discussion prior hysterectomy for potential sexual changes after surgery is crucial and may enhance the situation [36]. Another problem that might occur is the urinary problems after the operation or hysterectomy for sexually active and healthy women, they resulted in sexual dysfunction and increase in depression. The age, educational status, working condition and family structure is also important in this case [37].

In the other study, that is titled by" Women's attitudes about sexuality". In the third month after hysterectomy 49.5% of the women had begun to have sexual intercourse again, 34.3% of those were determined to have a decrease in sexual functions. It was also found that level of depression was less in the postoperative period compared to the preoperative period. Three months after hysterectomy, sexual functioning had significantly decreased. A clear resolution in symptoms of depression was seen after hysterectomy. It was determined that sexual functioning after hysterectomy was affected by advanced age, a women's attitude about sexuality, and the type of hysterectomy [28].

It is indicated in this review that sexual function is a major cause of women's concern for scheduled hysterectomy; therefore, it is important to spread awareness among women and let them know that most probably they will neither lose their sexual desire after hysterectomy, nor they will lose their feminine shape or style [26]. It is important to figure if ethnicity, socioeconomic status and sexual function are taken into account; it is easily to manage the physical and psychological changes [17].

3. Conclusion and recommendation

The health care profession should have insight regards the perception of women of her body after hystrectomy. In order to provide a competent health care for women based of her needs. Women's sexuality fractioning is essence and concern of women after hysterectomy, this topic is debated and controversial from literature. It is important here to highlight that uterus has symbolic values related to femininity as mentioned previously and evidence by many studies [38]. This problem among Arabian women is apparent and clear, where the womb of a woman is considered everything for her it represent it femininity and fertility, it means a lot for her. The woman inside herself felt of "deficient being" in the eyes of herself and her extended family, taking into consideration the presented of conservative culture that women's have and early marriage practice that aimed to protect women and produce more children from cultural lenses view. This leads us the significant to power women by increase her awareness pre-operative, follow up post-operative and having a good support system.

Educational programs for women undergoing hysterectomy will promote better self-care behavior, reduce postoperative anxiety and pain, and mitigate some of the negative influences of hysterectomy. So, interventions may not affect the actual incidence of the side-effects; they may help patients cope with adverse outcomes better, thus emphasizing the importance of the adaptation process to accept this condition with a positive thought.

The results of this review reveal that hysterectomy had significant argumentative effects on women's' quality of life, physically, psychological and sexually. For effective handling of this problem, healthcare profession must be aware of these potentially problematic issues and use effective intervention pre-post operation. Multidisciplinary teams have to work together, nurses have to lead the work to ensure of using the holistic approach that cover women's needs that included physical, psychological, spiritually, culturally and be individually. One size not fit all.

The important point here, that we could not change the culture or the mistake in the interpretation of religion. So, the practical solution is to involve the family into the therapeutic plan, identifying and addressing the psychosocial problems of the particularly high-risk groups is another critical point and referred them.

Based on the findings from this review, recommendations can be made to nurses working at gynecological departments. Nurses could also help the patients explore current coping mechanisms and support systems after hysterectomy. Another recommendation is to conduct a future study that examine the current education that provides to women pre-post operatively and it suitability based on her ethnicity and needs where ever the women is presented in her home country or diaspora.

Author details

Eman Alshawish
Head of Midwifery and MCH Department, Faculty of Medicine and Health Science, An-Najah National University, Nablus, Palestine

*Address all correspondence to: alshawish@najah.edu

References

[1] Kovac SR. Hysterectomy outcomes in patients with similar indications. Obstet Gynecol 2000; 95(6 Pt 1): 787-93. [PMID: 10831967]

[2] Spilsbury K Semmens JB Hammond I Bolck A. Persistent high rates of hysterectomy in Western Australia: a population-based study of 83 000 procedures over 23 years. BJOG: An International Journal of Obstetrics and Gynaecology 2006; 113: 804-9.

[3] Whiteman MK Hillis SD Jamieson DJ , et al. Inpatient hysterectomy surveillance in the United States, 2000-2004. American Journal of Obstetrics and Gynecology 2008; 198: 34 e1-7.

[4] Stankiewicz A Pogany L Popadiuk C. Prevalence of self-reported hysterectomy among Canadian women, 2000/2001-2008. Chronic Diseases and Injuries in Canada 2014; 34: 30-5.

[5] Carlson KJ Nichols DH Schiff I. Indications for hysterectomy. New England Journal of Medicine 1993; 328: 856-60.

[6] Dorsey JH, Steinberg EP, Holtz PM. Clinical indications for hysterectomy route: patient characteristics or physician preference? Am J Obstet Gynecol 1995; 173(5): 1452-60. [http://dx.doi.org/10.1016/0002-9378(95)90632-0] [PMID: 7503184]

[7] Matteson KA, Raker CA, Clark MA, Frick KD. Abnormal uterine bleeding, health status, and usual source of medical care: Analyses using the medical expenditures panel survey. J Womens Health (Larchmt) 2013;22:959-65. [PMC free article]

[8] Lis,Wagner.,Anne.,MetteCarls lund,Mette.,Sorensen,Bent.,Otte sen. Women's experience with short admission in abdominal hysterectomy and their patterns of behavior 2005; (19) :330-336.

[9] Valerie,Fleming. Hyserectomy a case study of one woman's experience 2003; 44(6): 575-582.

[10] Williams, R. and A. Clark. "A qualitative study of women's hysterectomy experience." Journal of women's health & gender-based medicine 9 Suppl 2 (2000): S15-25 .

[11] Gul Pinar, SeydaOkdem., NevinDogan, LaleBuyukgonec., Ali Ayhan. The effect of hysterectomy on body image self-esteem and marital adjustment in Turkish women with Gynecologic cancer 2011.

[12] Cara, Z.,delacruz , Martha,L.,Coul ter,Kathleen.,O'rourke,Aminaalio,Elle n,M Daley.,Charles ,S Mahan. Women's Experiences emotional responses and perceptions of care after emergency peripartum hysterectomy a Qualitative survery of women form 6 months to 3 years postpartum 2013.

[13] Uskulasye,K.,ahamd,farah.,Leyland, Nicholas.,A,sterwart,donna. Women's hysterectomy Experience and decision making 2003; 38 (1): 53-67

[14] DaugbjergSignem, B., cearoniGiulia, Ottesen bent, Diderichesn Finn, Osler Merete. Effect of socioeconomic position on patient outcome after hysterectomy 2014; 93(9): 926-934.

[15] Alshawish, E., Qadous, Sh., & Yamani, A. (2020). Experience of Palestinian women after hysterectomy using a descriptive phenomenological Study. *The Open Nursing Journal*, *14*(1),74-79. doi: 10.2174/1874434602014010074.

[16] GulizOnat,Bayram.,NevinSahin. Hystrectomy's psychosexual effects in Turkish Women, 2008; 26:149-158.

[17] Li ping wong., Kulenthran Arumugam. physical psychological and sexual effects in multi-ethnic

Malaysian women how have undergone hysterectomy 2012; 38:1095-1105.

[18] Muaygil, R. U. A. I. M. "Her Uterus, Her Medical Decision? Dismantling Spousal Consent for Medically Indicated Hysterectomies in Saudi Arabia," Cambridge Quarterly of Healthcare Ethics. Cambridge University Press 2018; 27(3):397-407. doi: 10.1017/S0963180117000780.

[19] islamweb.net . Ruling on the surgical removal of the uterus. 2020; Fatwa No: 296863. https://www.islamweb.org/en/fatwa/296863/ruling-on-the-surgical-removal-of-the-uterus

[20] Desai, S., Campbell, O. M., Sinha, T., Mahal, A., & Cousens, S. Incidence and determinants of hysterectomy in a low-income setting in Gujarat, India. Health Policy and Planning 2016; 32(1), 68-78.

[21] Kürek Eken M, İlhan G, Temizkan O, Çelik EE, Herkiloğlu D, Karateke A. The impact of abdominal and laparoscopic hysterectomies on women's sexuality and psychological condition. Turk J Obstet Gynecol 2016; 13(4): 196-202. [http://dx.doi.org/10.4274/tjod.71245] [PMID: 28913121]

[22] Farquhar CM, Steiner CA. Hysterectomy rates in the United States 1990-1997. Obstet Gynecol 2002; 99(2): 229-34. [PMID: 11814502]

[23] Lonnée-Hoffmann RA, Schei B, Eriksson NH. Sexual experience of partners after hysterectomy, comparing subtotal with total abdominal hysterectomy. Acta Obstet Gynecol Scand 2006; 85(11): 1389-94. [http://dx.doi.org/10.1080/00016340600917316] [PMID: 17091422]

[24] Mylonas I, Friese K. Indications for and Risks of Elective Cesarean Section. Dtsch Arztebl Int 2015; 112(29-30): 489-95. [http://dx.doi.org/10.3238/arztebl.2015.0489] [PMID: 26249251]

[25] Danesh M, Hamzehgardeshi Z, Moosazadeh M, Shabani-Asrami F. The Effect of Hysterectomy on Women's Sexual Function: a Narrative Review. Med Arh 2015; 69(6): 387-92.[http://dx.doi.org/10.5455/medarh.2015.69.387-392] [PMID: 26843731]

[26] Fram KM, Saleh SS, Sumrein IA. Sexuality after hysterectomy at University of Jordan Hospital: a teaching hospital experience. Arch Gynecol Obstet 2013; 287(4): 703-8. [http://dx.doi.org/10.1007/s00404-012-2601-2] [PMID: 23132049]

[27] Goetsch MF. The effect of total hysterectomy on specific sexual sensations. Am J Obstet Gynecol 2005; 192(6): 1922-7. [http://dx.doi.org/10.1016/j.ajog.2005.02.065] [PMID: 15970852]

[28] Bayram., NevinSahin. Hystrectomy's Psychosexual Effects in Turkish Women 2008; 26: 149-58.

[29] Lonnée-Hoffmann R, Pinas I. Effects of Hysterectomy on Sexual Function. Curr Sex Health Rep 2014; 6(4): 244-51. [http://dx.doi.org/10.1007/s11930-014-0029-3] [PMID: 25999801]

[30] Farquhar CM, Steiner CA. Hysterectomy rates in the United States 1990-1997. Obstet Gynecol 2002; 99(2): 229-34. [PMID: 11814502]

[31] Altman D, Granath F, Cnattingius S, Falconer C. Hysterectomy and risk of stress-urinary-incontinence surgery: nationwide cohort study. Lancet 2007; 370(9597): 1494-9.[http://dx.doi.org/10.1016/S0140-6736(07)61635-3] [PMID: 17964350]

[32] Pauls RN. Impact of gynecological surgery on female sexual function. Int J Impot Res 2010; 22(2): 105-14.[http://dx.doi.org/10.1038/ijir.2009.63] [PMID: 20072131]

[33] Adorna E, Morari-Cassol E, Ferraz N. A Mastectomia e suas

Repercussões na Vida Afetiva, Familiar e Social da Mulher. Rev Saúde (Santa Maria) 2017; 43(1): 163-8.

[34] Schmidt, Alessandra, Sehnem, Graciela Dutra, Cardoso, Leticia Silveira, Quadros, Jacqueline Silveira de, Ribeiro, Aline Cammarano, & Neves, Eliane Tatsch. Sexuality experiences of hysterectomized women. Ginekol Pol Esc Anna Nery 2019; 23(4)

[35] G So, sozeri-varma., N kalkan – Oguzbanolgu ,F., Karadag , gand O.Ozdel. The effect of hysterectomy and oophorectomy on sexual satisfaction 2011;14: 275-281.

[36] Meston CM, Bradford A. Sexual dysfunctions in women. Annu Rev Clin Psychol. 2007;3:233-56. doi: 10.1146/ annurev.clinpsy.3.022806.091507. PMID: 17716055.

[37] Goktas SB, Gun I, Yildiz T, Sakar MN, Caglayan S. The effect of total hysterectomy on sexual function and depression. Pak J Med Sci. 2015;31(3):700-5. doi: 10.12669/ pjms.313.7368. PMID: 26150871; PMCID: PMC4485298.

[38] Silva CMC, Vargens OMC. A mulher que vivencia as cirurgias ginecológicas: enfrentando as mudanças impostas pelas cirurgias. Rev Latino-Am Enferm 2016; 24(e2780): 1-8.